Special Veterinary Pathology

NIPA® GENX ELECTRONIC RESOURCES & SOLUTIONS P. LTD.
New Delhi-110 034

About the Authors

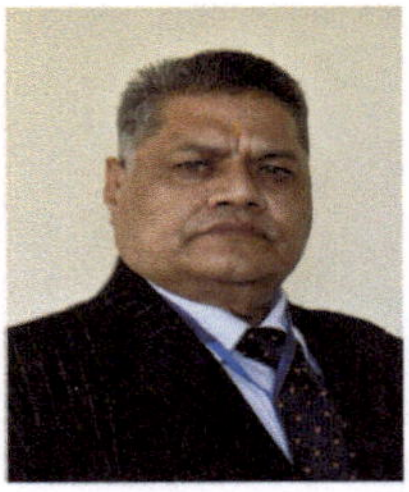

Prof RS Chauhan – Cowpathy Man, MVSc, PhD, FNAVS FSIIP, FIAVP, Diplomat ICVP, PDCR, ACPPM, OCTT MBA EX- Director ICAR-IVRI, JD CADRAD, Director IBT National Fellow, Advisor WHO. Member, Animal Welfare Board of India; Member, CPCSEA (Govt. of India); Chairman Scientific Advisory Committee, ICMR-NARFBR.

Born on September 10th, 1958 in a farmer's family, Dr. Chauhan completed his Bachelors (80.3%) with honours, Master (85.8%) and Doctoral degree (90.0%) in Veterinary Sciences with specialization in veterinary pathology from G.B. Pant University of Agric. & Tech., Pantnagar. He served the country in various capacities including Assistant Professor/ADIO (1983-96), Associate Professor (1996-1999), National Fellow (1999-2004) and Joint Director (CADRAD), IVRI, Izatnagar(2004-2009), Director & Vice-Chancellor(2009), ICAR-IVRI and Campus Director, IBT, Patwadangar (2009-2013). During his tenure as academician and scientist, he has written 112 books including 35 manuals and 1 monograph very popular among the students world over. He contributed 99 chapters in different books and published 235 research and 59 review papers. Besides, he participated in International / National Conferences and presented 178 papers. He is life member of 15 scientific bodies and has been in several executive committee such as Chairman, Panch Gavya Professionals' Club; President, Cow Therapy Society; Secretary-General, Society for Immunology and Immunopathology; Vice President, Indian Society of Veterinary Educators; Zonal Secretary, Indian Association of Veterinary Pathologists and Joint Secretary, Indian Virology Society, President, Dr. J.L. Vegad Foundation, Expert Member Research Group, Committee for Certification of Pathologists, Vice-President, IAVP; Registrar, ICVP, etc.

Based on his contributions and scientific achievements, he has been awarded with several prizes, medals and honours including Best Young Scientist Award (1992), IAAVR Award (1996), National Fellow Award (1999), Fellow NAVS (2000), Fellow SIIP (2001), K.S. Nair Memorial Award (1999), Vigyan Bharti Award (2000), Dr. C.M. Singh Trust Award (2002), Dr. Rajendra Prasad Award (2002), Shri Ramlal Agrawal National Award (2000), Best Paper Award SIIP (2003), Best Paper Award IAVA (2001, 2002, 2003), Best Teacher Award (2004) by GBPUAT, Fellow, IAVP (2006), Gopal Gaurav (2007), Bharat Excellence Award (2007), Diplomat, ICVP (2008), Intas-ISVE Best Veterinary Scientist Award (2008), Best Academician Award (2012), Moropant Pingle Go Sewa National Award (2015), Outstanding Scientist Award (2019), Research Excellence Award (2020), Indo

Asian-Claude Bourgelat Distinguished Innovative Scientist Award-2020 in Animal Immunopathology and MAN OF COWPATHY at GADVASU Ludhiana etc. in recognition of his research and teaching endeavor. He has been inducted in many national and international scientific/advisory committees and boards including Member, WHO/IPCS Committee on Environmental Health Criteria. Dr. Chauhan added many new including Enterotoxaemia, Pyometra, ETEC infection in camels, isolated camel pox virus, developed rapid diagnostic test DIA for the first time in India. He reported role of cell mediated immunity in rotavirus infection in calves. His pioneer work includes immunopathology due to pesticides, heavy metals, mycotoxins and nanoparticles. Dr. Chauhan developed a new method using MTT dye for detection of CMI response. He has scientifically validated Panchgavya and named it as "Cowpathy".

He have been recognized internationally as visiting Professor, University of Wageningen and Advisor, WHO. Dr. Chauhan guided more than 50 scholars for their Masters and Doctoral research; most of them are placed as Professors, Scientists, Officers in Indian Army, banks and industry in India and abroad. At present he is working as Head Veterinary Pathology, Chairman Scientific Advisory Committee ICMR-NARFBR, Member AWBI and CPCSEA (Govt of India). Prof Chauhan superannuated on 30th June 2024 after distinguish service of 41.5 years and still contributing to the profession through lectures, writings and research and particularly developing literature/ books for the benefit of students and young generation.

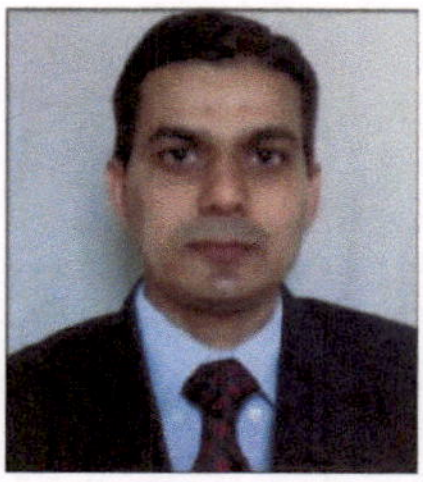

Prof. (Dr.) Desh Deepak Singh is Veterinary Graduate and Post Graduate in Veterinary Pathology from College of Veterinary and Animal Sciences, Govind Ballabh Pant University of Agriculture and Technology (GBPUA&T), Pantnagar (Uttarakhand) India in 2001 and 2003. He was awarded outstanding PG student award by GBPUA&T, Pantnagar in 2003. He visited Istanbul, Turkey to present research paper in world poultry congress-2004. He joined as Assistant Professor, Department of Veterinary Pathology, College of Veterinary Sciences & Animal Husbandry, Acharya Narendra Dev University of Agriculture & Technology (ANDUA&T), Kumarganj, Ayodhya, Uttar Pradesh in 2004. He completed his Ph.D. as in-service candidate from U. P. Pandit Deen Dayal Upadhyaya Pashu Chikitsa Vigyan Vishwavidyalaya Evam Go Anusandhan Sansthan (DUVASU), Mathura, Uttar Pradesh, India and promoted to Associate Professor in ANDUA&T, Kumarganj, Ayodhya. Prof. Singh was selected as Professor, Veterinary Pathology, DUVASU, Mathura and presently working as Professor & Head, Veterinary Pathology, DUVASU, Mathura. He is having more than 20 years' experience of teaching Undergraduate (UG) and Postgraduate (PG) courses of Veterinary Pathology along with vast experience of disease diagnosis, research and extension. He has published more than 55 original research papers in referred journals, 04 books, 04 laboratory manuals for Under Graduate students, 02 manuals for Veterinary Officers, 08 review articles, 10 book chapters and 54 technical/popular articles. He was awarded young scientist award by Society of Immunology and Immunopathology; Prakash best poster award; best poster award by Indian Association of Veterinary Pathology (IAVP); best paper presentation award by Indian Society of Veterinary Anatomy; best poster award by UP chapter of Indian Society of Veterinary Surgery; best paper award in National Conference held at ANDUA&T, Kumarganj, Ayodhya, Uttar Pradesh; Best poster and best oral presentation award by Indian Society of Veterinary Pharmacology and Toxicology (ISVPT). Prof. Singh is life member of Indian Association of Veterinary Pathologists (IAVP) since 2002; Society of Immunology and Immunopathology (SIIP), Indian Association of Veterinary Public Health Specialists (IAVPHS)..

Special Veterinary Pathology
(Pathology of Infectious and Non-infectious Diseases of Domestic, Pet, Laboratory and Wild Animals)

R.S. Chauhan
M.V.Sc., Ph.D. (Path.), FNAVS, FSIIP, FIAVP, PDCR, OCTT, ACPPM, MBA
(Ex- Advisor WHO, Ex- Director IVRI, Ex-JDCADRAD, Ex-Director IBT,
Ex- National Fellow ICAR)
Member Animal Welfare Board of India (Govt. of India)
Member, CCSEA (Govt of India)
Chairman, SAC, NARFBR (ICMR)
Ex-Professor and Head, Department of Veterinary Pathology
GB Pant University of Agriculture & Technology Pantnagar - 263 145
Uttarakhand, India

Desh Deepak Singh
M.V.Sc., Ph.D.
Professor & Head
Department of Veterinary Pathology
U. P. Pandit Deen Dayal Upadhyaya Pashu Chikitsa Vigyan Vishwavidyalaya Evam
Go Anusandhan, Sansthan (DUVASU), Mathura-281001, Uttar Pradesh, India

NIPA® GENX ELECTRONIC RESOURCES & SOLUTIONS P. LTD.
New Delhi-110 034

NIPA® GENX ELECTRONIC
RESOURCES & SOLUTIONS P. LTD.

101,103, Vikas Surya Plaza, CU Block
L.S.C.Market, Pitam Pura, New Delhi-110 034
Ph : +91 11 4386 0225, 9717133558, 9540816132
E-mail: newindiapublishingagency@gmail.com
Website: www.niparesources.com

Print ISBN: 978-93-5887-980-3

ebook ISBN: 978-93-5887-778-6

Composed and Designed by NIPA®.

Preface

Veterinary Pathology is an important discipline of Veterinary Sciences which makes a bridge in between the basic and clinical sciences. The knowledge of Veterinary Pathology makes the Veterinarian a perfect diagnostician particularly when his patients (animal) can't speak their illness to the doctor. Keeping in view the need of study of Veterinary Pathology to become a good Veterinary doctor, the book "Special Veterinary Pathology (Pathology of infectious and non-infectious diseases of domestic, pet, laboratory and wild animals)" is written for the use of teachers, students and field veterinarians. The complexity of the subject is presented in a simplified way particularly keeping the view of Indian geo-climatic conditions and animal population. However, students of Veterinary Science desire a compact text of Special Veterinary Pathology (Pathology of infectious and non-infectious diseases of domestic, pet, laboratory and wild animals) covering the VCI new syllabus of pathology which can be utilized during their study and examinations particularly in competitive examinations. Hence, this textbook is prepared as a text material to all those who want to know Special Veterinary Pathology (Pathology of infectious and non-infectious diseases of domestic, pet, laboratory and wild animals) at undergraduate and postgraduate level and are interested in any kind of competitive examination or interview. It covers all the topics of Pathology of infectious and non-infectious diseases of domestic, pet, laboratory and wild animals. The text is described in a very simple format including pathology of bacterial; viral; chlamydial; rickettsial; mycoplasmal; spirochaetal; prion; fungal; parasitic; nutritional and metabolic disorders; toxicopathology; diseases of laboratory and wild animals including their etiology, clinical manifestations, characteristic macroscopic and microscopic features along with diagnosis; only salient features are mentioned avoiding detailed text. Hope this book "Special Veterinary Pathology (Pathology of infectious and non-infectious diseases of domestic, pet, laboratory and wild animals)" not only will find a place in the young fraternity of Veterinary Science but also it will be highly useful to the field Veterinarians for diagnosing diseases on the basis of characteristic clinical manifestations, and lesions and in writing of post mortem report. The help rendered by our colleagues and students in preparation and designing of this book is duly acknowledged. Readers' comments are welcome to further improve the book

R.S. Chauhan
D.D. Singh

Contents

1

Pathology of Viral Diseases

Foot and Mouth disease

Foot and mouth disease is a contagious viral disease of cloven footed animals caused by a picorna virus and characterized by presence of vesicles in oral mucosa and foot (Fig.1.1).

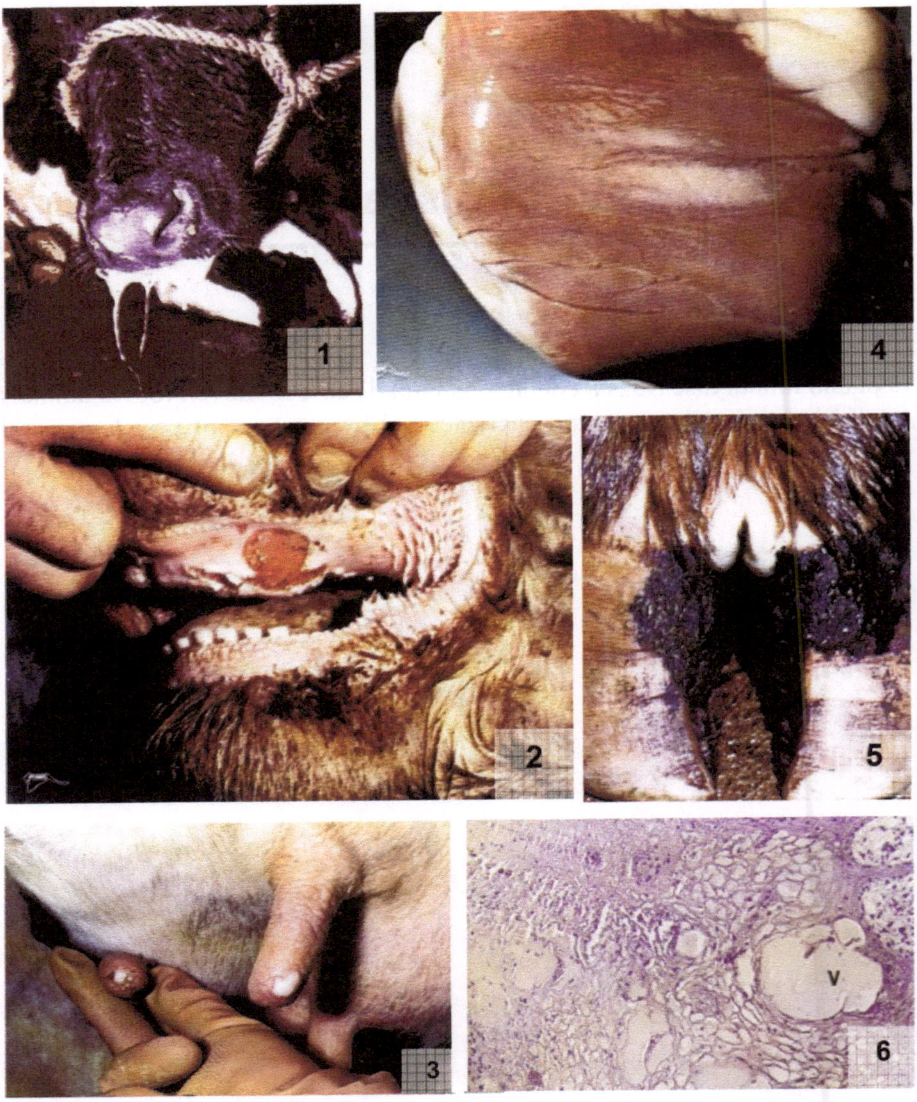

Fig. 1.1: Foot and mouth disease in cattle- (1) Hypersalivation (2) Ruptured vesicle in hard palate (3) Vesicle on teats (4) Tigroid appearance on heart (5) Presence of vesicles on coronets and (6) Microscopic picture of mucous membrane having vesicle.

Etiology

- RNA virus of picornaviridae family
- Picorna virus
- Serotypes A,O,C, SAT-1, SAT-2, SAT-3, Asia-1, serotype 'O' is most common in India.

Pathogenesis

Inhalation is the main route of infection in ruminants; however, ingestion of contaminated feed and water, inoculation of contaminated vaccines, insemination with contaminated semen and contact with fomites such as clothing, instruments etc. may also transmit the infection. When animal gets infected through respiratory tract, viral replication starts in pharynx followed by viraemic spread to other tissues and organs like epithelium of mouth. Viral excretion commences about 24 hours prior to the onset of clinical form of disease and continues for several days. The aerosols of infected animals contain large amount of virus particularly of swine. Large amount of virus is excreted in milk. In cattle and sheep, virus may be detectable up to 2 years and 6 months of exposure, respectively.

Characteristic symptoms

- Fever(102-104°F)
- Drooling of saliva
- Vesicular mouth lesions
- Lameness due to formation of vesicles on coronets

Macroscopic features

- Presence of vesicles on tongue, lips, cheeks and palate
- Damaged vesicle leaves a raw surface having red areas due to congestion
- Gastroenteritis
- Myocarditis- ***Tigroid appearance***
- Enlargement of spleen.

Microscopic features

- Hydropic degeneration in stratum spinosum cells of epidermis
- Presence of micro vesicles

- Infiltration of neutrophils
- Hyaline degeneration and necrosis of muscles of myocardium
- Infiltration of neutrophils and mononuclear cells in myocardium.

Diagnosis

- Symptoms and lesions
- Immunodiagnostic tests for demonstration of antigen /antibody
- CFT
- ELISA
- Isolation of virus and its typing
- Demonstration of virus in affected tissues using electronmicroscopy

Vesicular Stomatitis

Vesicular stomatitis is a contagious viral disease of animals caused by vesiculovirus and characterized by the presence of vesicles in oral cavity, necrosis and intercellular oedema. It is also known as ***sore mouth*** of cattle (Fig.1.2).

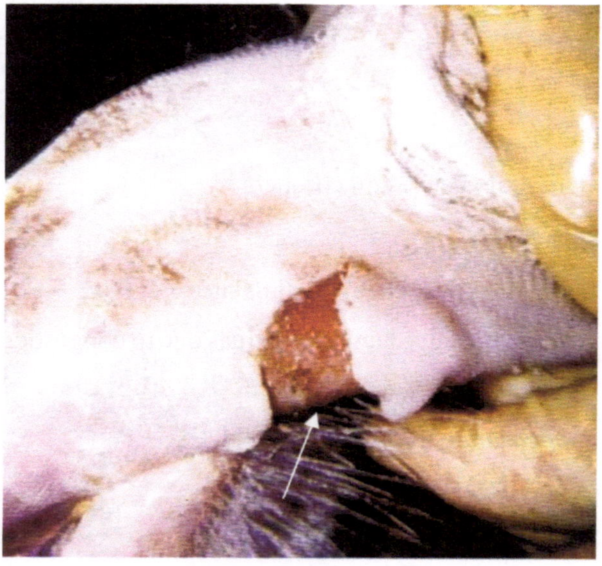

Fig. 1.2: Vesicular stomatitis ruptured vesicle on tongue (arrow).

Etiology

- Vesiculovirus of rhabdoviridae family.
- RNA virus with 70-175 nm size, bullet shape

Pathogenesis

Transmitted through insects from infected to susceptible animals. There is viraemia and virus settles in oral mucosa causing vesicular glossitis.

Clinical Symptoms

- Hypersalivation
- Rubbing of lips with manger

Macroscopic features

- Vesicles on tongue
- Vesicles on snout of pigs

Microscopic features

- Intercellular oedema in malpighian layer
- Necrosis of epithelial layer
- Infiltration of neutrophils and mononuclear cells

Diagnosis

- Symptoms and lesions
- Detection of antibody or antigen using ELISA

Vesicular Exanthema

Vesicular exanthema is a viral disease of swine characterized by fever and vesicle formation in snout, lips, nostrils, tongue, feet and mammary gland (Fig.1.3).

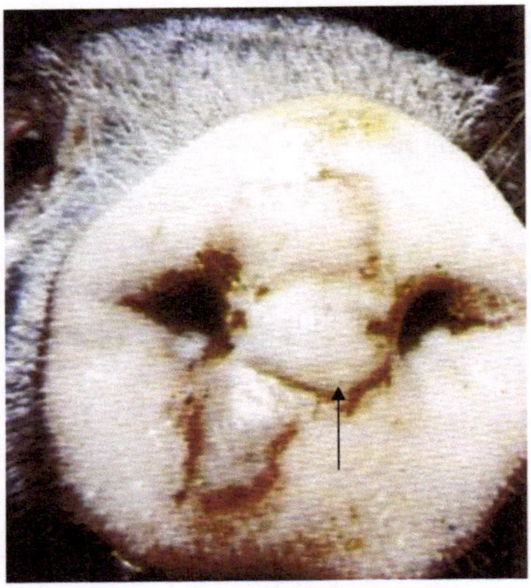

Fig. 1.3: Vesicular exanthema- vesicle on snout (arrow)

Etiology

- Calcivirus of 35-40 nm diameter

Pathogenesis

The source of infection is infected pig or pork and virus spreads among susceptible animals through direct contact. Viraemia lasts for 3-4 days and virus localizes in buccal mucosa and skin.

Clinical Symptoms

- Fever
- Vesicles on mouth, snout, teats, claws
- Anorexia
- Rupture of vesicle leads to ulcer

Macroscopic features

- Vesicles on snouts, lips, tongue
- Vesicles on coronary band and mammary gland
- Rupture of vesicles
- Ruptured vesicles covered by brown and dry dead tissue
- Ulcer on secondary bacterial infection.

Microscopic features

- Vesicles, hydropic degeneration on stratum spinosum layer of epidermis
- Infiltration of mononuclear cells

Diagnosis

- Symptoms and lesions
- Detection of antibody or antigen using ELISA

Rinderpest

Rinderpest is an acute contagious viral disease of cattle and buffaloes caused by morbilli virus and characterized by erosive mouth lesions and erosions and hemorrhagic enteritis. It has been eradicated from India (Fig.1.4).

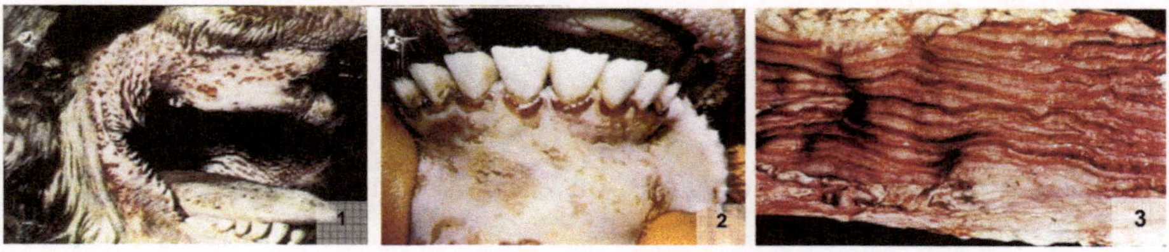

Fig. 1.4: Rinderpest in buffaloes- (1) Erosions on hard palate (2) Gums and (3) Zebra stripping on large intestines.

Etiology

- Morbilli virus of paramyxoviridae family.
- RNA virus
- Very fragile virus, sensitive to glycerol.

Pathogenesis

Virus enters in body through inhalation, penetrates the epithelium of upper respiratory tract and multiplies in tonsils and mandibular and pharyngeal lymph nodes. From there it enters in blood mononuclear cells, which disseminate the virus to other lymphoid organs, lungs and epithelial cells of mucous membrane. The virus has high affinity for lymphoid tissue and alimentary tract mucosa. In tissues, there is pronounced destruction of lymphocytes. Viremia develops within 2 to 3 days after which virus can be demonstrated in lymph nodes, spleen, bone marrow and mucosa of respiratory and digestive tract. There is marked leucopenia due to viral replication and destruction of lymphoid tissue.

Due to destruction of epithelial lining of mucous membranes, there is presence of erosions in the form of "Zebra" stripes in caecum, colon and rectum which is considered characteristic of rinderpest. Intra cytoplasmic and intra nuclear eosinophilic inclusion bodies are commonly seen in epithelial cells.

Characteristic symptoms

- Fever(105-107°F)
- Diarrhoea, melena
- Erosive mouth lesions
- Skin eruptions
- Conjunctivitis
- Mortality up to 80%

Macroscopic features

- Erosions on oral mucosa
- Bran like deposits on erosions, on removal hemorrhagic raw surface is present
- Hemorrhage in intestines leading to "***Zebra markings***"
- Petechial hemorrhage in bladder, vagina and other mucous membrane
- Congestion of conjunctivae.

Microscopic features

- Erosions in epithelium of oral and gastrointestinal mucosa
- Infiltration of mononuclear cells
- Congestion and hemorrhage in intestines
- Depletion of lymphoid cells in Peyer's patches
- Lymphocytolysis in spleen and lymph nodes.

Diagnosis

- Symptoms and lesions
- Immunodiagnostic tests for demonstration of antigen /antibody
- AGPT
- CIEP

- ELISA
- Isolation of virus

Malignant Catarrhal Fever

Malignant catarrhal fever is an infectious disease of cattle caused by herpes virus and characterized by catarrhal and mucopurulent conjunctivitis, presence of erosions / ulcers on nostrils, oral mucosa, intestines and enlargement of lymph nodes (Fig.1.5).

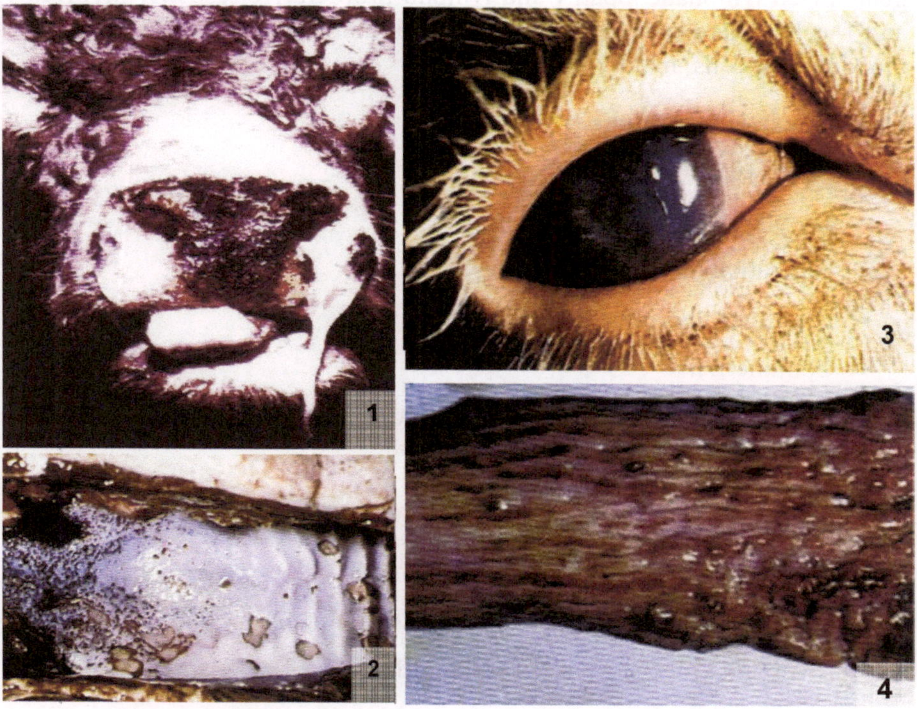

Fig. 1.5: Malignant catarrhal fever- (1) Tenacious nasal discharge, (2) Ulcers on oral mucosa, (3) Opacity in eye and (4) Ulcers and zebra stripping on intestine.

Etiology

- DNA virus of herpesviridae family
- Herpes virus

Pathogenesis

It is caused by herpes virus which is strongly associated with cells. The disease is transmitted through wild beast and sub clinically infected sheep to cattle. In circulating blood it is attached to leucocytes, especially mononuclear cells. After entry, the virus attacks and replicates in lymphoid tissues (e.g. lymph nodes, Peyer's patches and spleen). Many lymphocytes are destroyed in germinal centers leading to their depletion. The incubation period is very long and there is no clear information about pathogenesis of disease. There is generalized lymphadenopathy and lympho-proliferative response involves T_h and T_c cells. There is most constant finding is marked perivascular coughing of mononuclear cells, mainly monocytes.

Characteristic symptoms

- Fever(105-107°F)
- Drooling of saliva
- Ulcerative mouth and nasal lesions
- Diarrhoea, dysentery with melena
- Conjunctivitis
- Enlargement of superficial lymph nodes

Macroscopic features

- Conjunctivitis, rhinitis
- Mucopurulent exudate in eyes and nostrils
- Erosions and ulcers on oral and intestinal mucosa
- Liver and kidneys enlarged and mottled

Microscopic features

- Necrosis of epithelium and intense lymphocytic infiltration in mucosa of upper respiratory tract, oral mucosa and abomasum
- Infiltration of eosinophils in mucosa and sub mucosa of gastrointestinal tract.

Diagnosis

- History of sheep rearing with cattle
- Symptoms and lesions

- Immunodiagnostic tests for demonstration of antigen /antibody
- AGPT
- ELISA
- Isolation of virus through co-cultivation of peripheral blood lymphocytes

Bovine Viral Diarrhoea / Mucosal Disease

Bovine viral diarrhoea is a contagious viral disease of cattle caused by pestivirus and characterized by hypoplasia of cerebellum, ulcers in oral and nasal mucosa, oesophagus, abomasum and intestines (Fig.1.6).

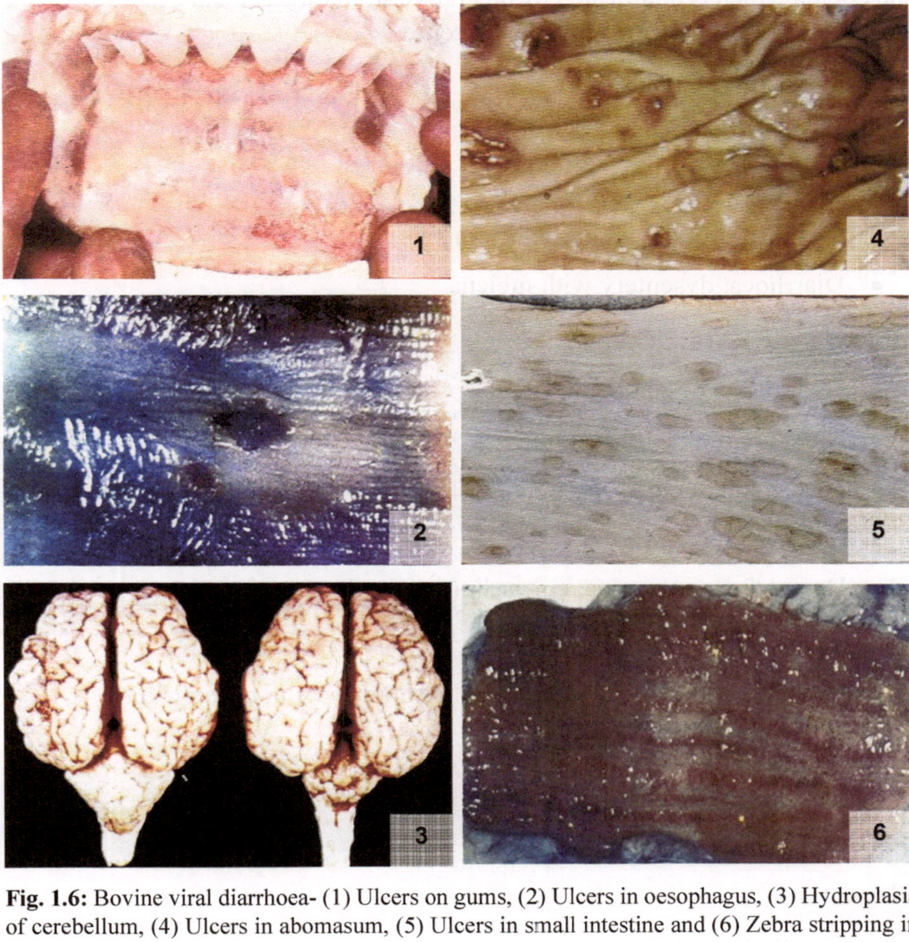

Fig. 1.6: Bovine viral diarrhoea- (1) Ulcers on gums, (2) Ulcers in oesophagus, (3) Hydroplasia of cerebellum, (4) Ulcers in abomasum, (5) Ulcers in small intestine and (6) Zebra stripping in large intestine.

Etiology

- Pestivirus of Togaviridae family.

Pathogenesis

The virus spreads by direct or indirect contact with infected animals. Overcrowding and transportation play an important role in spread of virus through oral and nasal route. The virus also spreads through contaminated food and water, urine and nasal discharge. After entry virus multiplies in lymphocytes which leads to viraemia. From circulation, virus reaches in the mucous membrane of alimentary tract. In buccal cavity, it causes inflammation and edema which is manifested by ulcerative stomatitis and enteritis. However, pathogenesis of the lesions remains obscure.

Characteristic symptoms

- Fever(105-107°F)
- Drooling of saliva
- Ulcerative mouth and nasal lesions
- Diarrhoea, dysentery with melena

Macroscopic features

- Hypoplasia of cerebellum
- Ulcers in oral and nasal mucosa
- Ulcers and hemorrhage in mucosa of gastrointestinal tract
- Ulcers in esophagus
- Hemorrhage in vagina, epicardium and sub cutaneous tissue.

Microscopic features

- Necrosis, ulcer, and infiltration of lymphocytes in oesophagus.
- Hemorrhage in intestines
- Ulcers in intestines
- Infiltration of mononuclear cells

Diagnosis

- Symptoms and lesions
- Immunodiagnostic tests for demonstration of antigen /antibody

- AGPT
- ELISA
- Isolation of virus

Pox

Pox is an infectious viral disease of animals caused by members of poxviridae family and characterized by the presence of pock lesions on hair less parts of the skin (Fig.1.7- Fig.1.10).

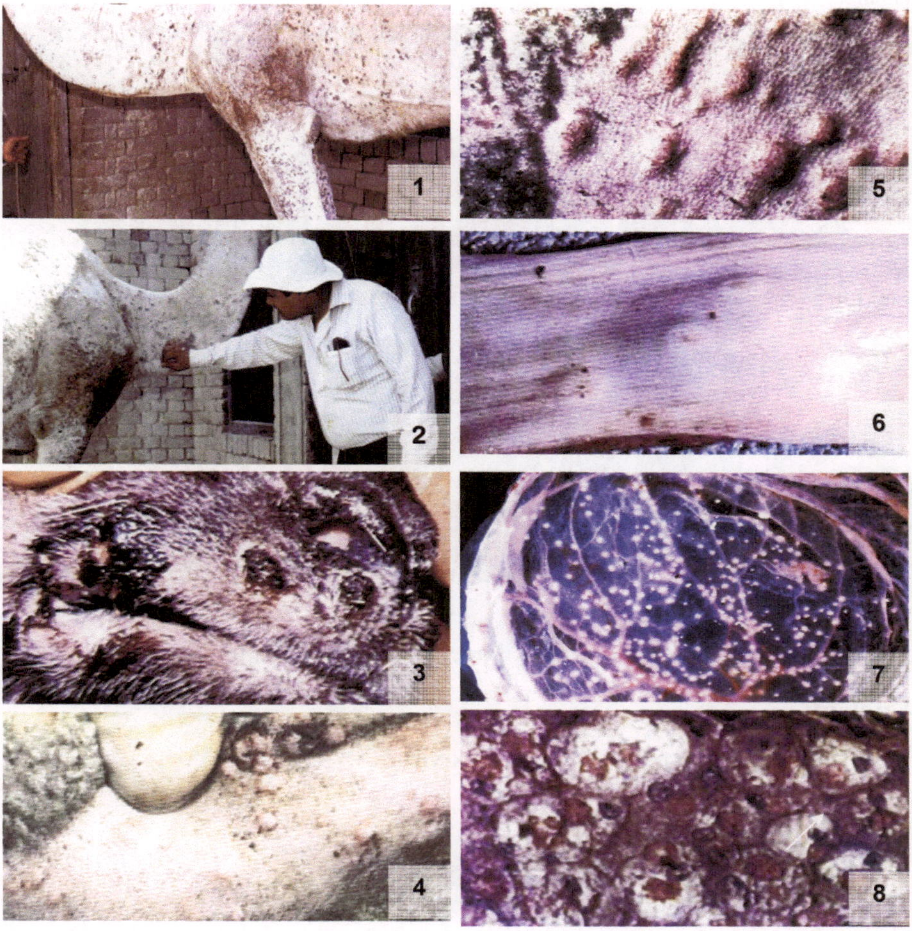

Fig. 1.7: Pox in animals- (1&2) Camel pox (3) Sheep pock lesions lips, (4) Pock lesions on beneath the tail, (5) Papules on ventral abdomen, (6) Pock lesions on oesophagus, (7) Pock lesions on CAM of developing chicken embryo and (8) Intracytoplasmic eosinophilic inclusions (arrow).

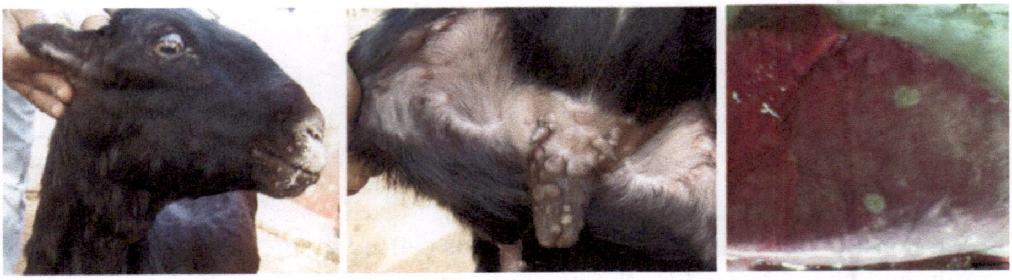

A **B** **C**

Fig. 1.8: Goat pox-A. Pock lesions at face and neck, B. Pock lesions at teat and C.Pock lesions in lung.

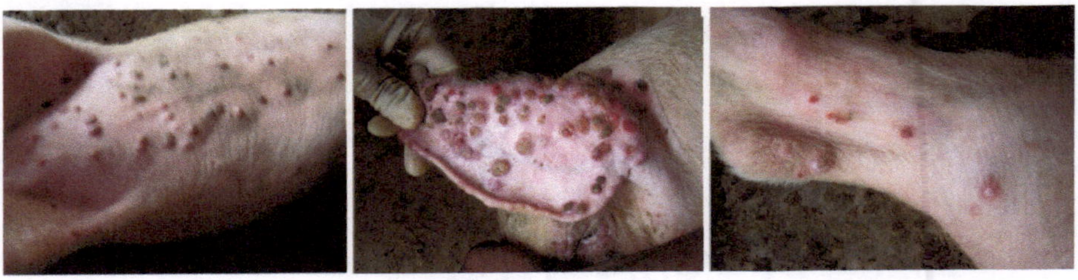

A **B** **C**

Fig. 1.9: Swine pox lesions at A. Belly, B. Ear and Legs.

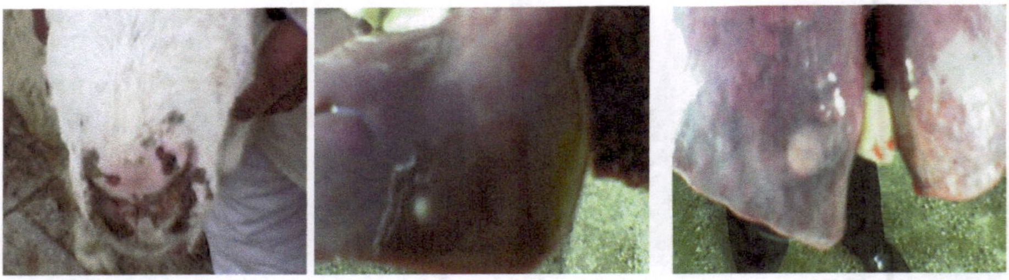

A B C

Fig. 1.10: Sheep pox lesions at A. Face, B. Liver and C. lungs.

Etiology

- Sheep - Ovi pox virus, Capri pox virus
- Goat - Capri pox virus
- Cow - Cow pox virus
- Buffalo - Buffalo pox virus
- Camel - Camel pox virus
- Swine - Swi pox virus

Pathogenesis

The disease is transmitted by direct contact with affected animals and through the hand of the milkers, insects and milking machine. Generally virus enters through small abrasions of skin. Following incubation period of 3-7 days, the pock lesions appear on skin which comprises of erythema, followed by papules, vesicles, pustule and scab; on detach and slough off it may leave scar.

Characteristic symptoms

- Fever(105-107°F)
- Pock lesions on hairless parts of skin like papule, vesicle, pustule, scab and scar

Macroscopic features

- Presence of pock lesions on hair less parts of body including papule, vesicle, pustule, scab and scar.
- Cow- Pock lesions on teats
- Buffaloes- Face, teats
- Sheep and Camel- Whole body

Microscopic features

- Necrosis of stratum spinosum epithelium of epidermis
- Infiltration of mononuclear cells in dermis and epidermis
- Presence of intracytoplasmic inclusions

Diagnosis

- Symptoms and lesions
- Immunodiagnostic tests for demonstration of antigen /antibody
- AGPT
- ELISA
- Isolation of virus

Infectious Bovine Rhinotracheitis

Infectious bovine rhinotracheitis is an infectious viral disease of cattle caused by herpes virus and characterized by respiratory disease, conjunctivitis, encephalitis in calves and abortions and mastitis in cows (Fig.1.11- Fig.1.12).

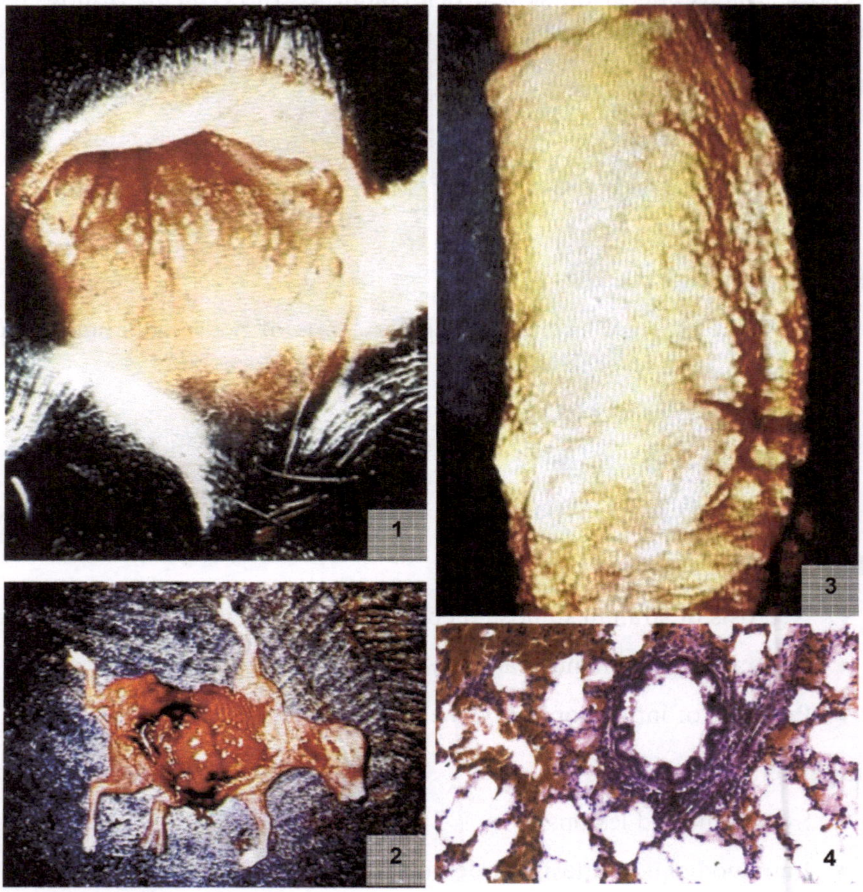

Fig. 1.11: Bovine herpes virus-1 infection in cattle- (1) Granular vaginititis, (2) Aborted foetus, (3) Granular balaeno-posthitis and (4) Hyaline membrane bronchopneumonia in aborted foetus

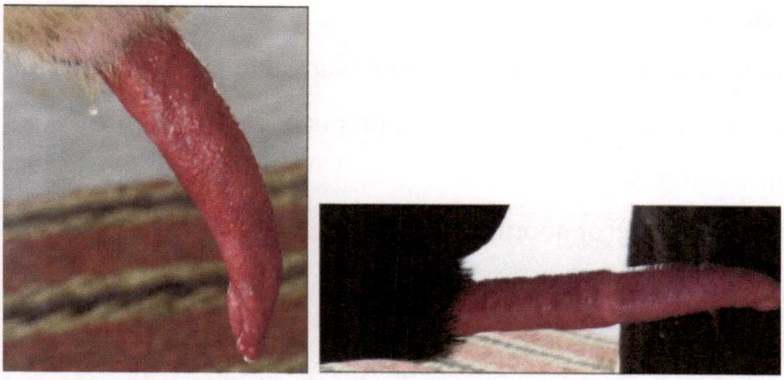

Fig. 1.12: BHV-1 infection in bulls-pustular balanoposthitis

Etiology

- DNA virus of Herpesviridae family
- Bovine herpes virus –1 (BHV-1)

Pathogenesis

The main source of infection is nasal exudate and coughed up droplets, genital secretions, semen and foetal fluid/ tissues. Aerosol or droplet infection causes respiratory disease. In genital from, venereal transmission occurs. In respiratory disease, after entry virus multiplies in nasal cavity and upper respiratory tract resulting in rhinitis, laryngitis and tracheitis. There is extensive loss of cilia in trachea. This leaves the tracheal epithelium covered with microvilli, which has an adverse effect on the defense mechanism of respiratory tract. The virus spreads from nasal mucosa through trigeminal ganglion, resulting in a non-suppurative encephalitis. Through peripheral leucocytes, virus may reach to placenta and foetus in pregnant animals causing abortion. The foetus is highly susceptible to the herpes virus infection.

Characteristic symptoms

- Fever(106°F)
- Nasal discharge
- Abortions in late gestation
- Conjunctivitis
- Infectious pustular balanoposthitis in bulls
- Infectious pustular vulvovaginitis in cows

Macroscopic features

- Rhinotracheitis, pneumonia, mucopurulent exudate in trachea.
- Pustules in vulva/vagina, glans penis and prepuce
- Ulcers in vulva/vagina
- Necrotic lesions in liver of aborted foetus

Microscopic features

- Hyaline membrane pneumonia
- Erosions/ulcers in mucosa of upper respiratory tract
- Ulcers on vulval mucous membrane
- Infiltration of lymphocytes
- Presence of intranuclear inclusions in mucosal epithelium
- Necrotic lesions in liver, spleen and kidneys of aborted foetus

Diagnosis

- Symptoms and lesions
- Immunodiagnostic tests for demonstration of antigen /antibody
- AGPT
- ELISA
- Isolation of virus

Rotavirus Infection

Rotavirus causes acute gastroenteritis in neonates of animals characterized by yellowish watery diarrhoea, shortening of villi, dehydration, malabsorption and mal digestion (Fig.1.13-Fig.1.15).

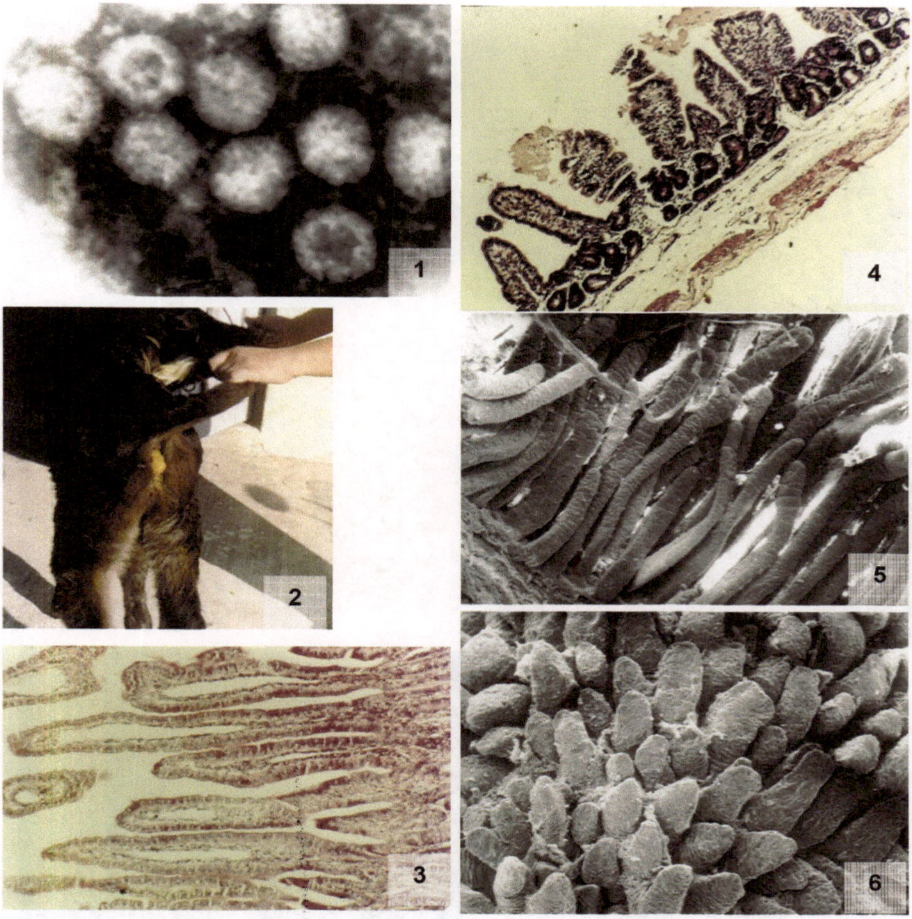

Fig. 1.13: Rotavirus infection in calves- (1) Rotavirus, (2) Yellowish diarrhoea in calf, (3) Elongated normal villi, (4) Short villi of calf infected with rotavirus,(5) Scanning electronic microscopic picture of normal villi, (6) Rotavirus infected villi.

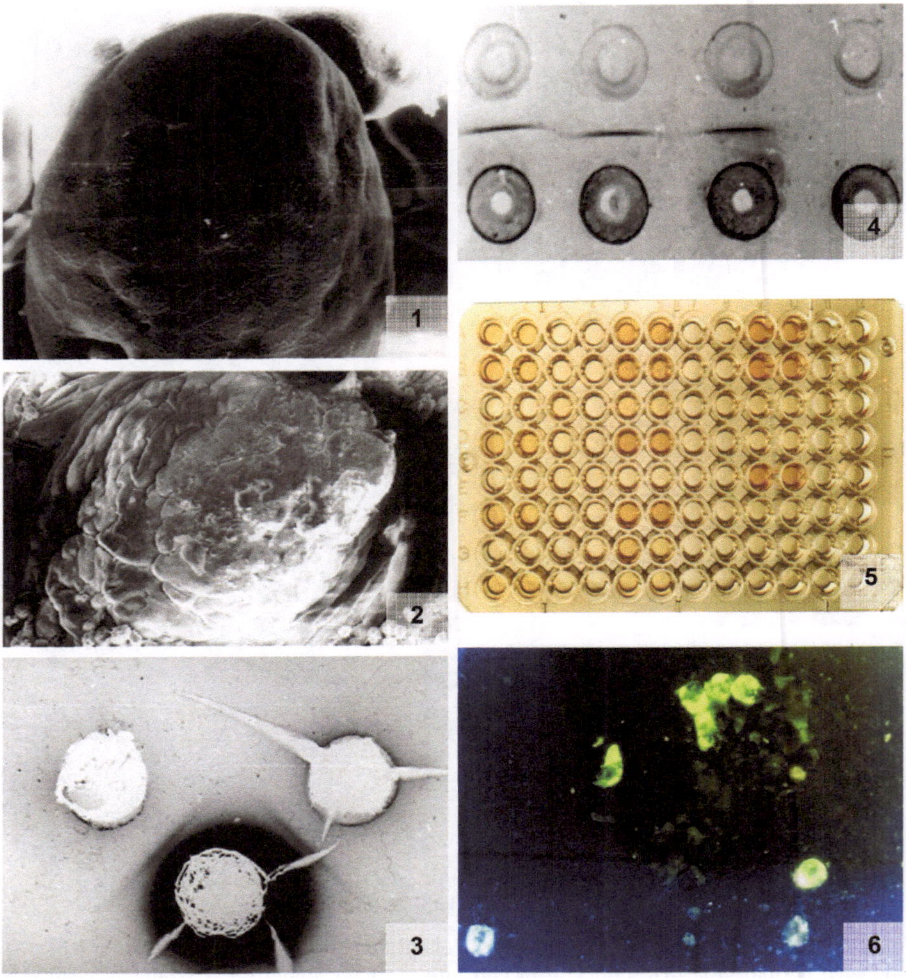

Fig. 1.14: Rotavirus infection in calves- (1) Scanning electronic microscopic picture of tip of normal villi, (2) Tip of infected villi, (3) AGPT, (4) CIEP, (5) ELISA and (6) Immunofluorescence assay.

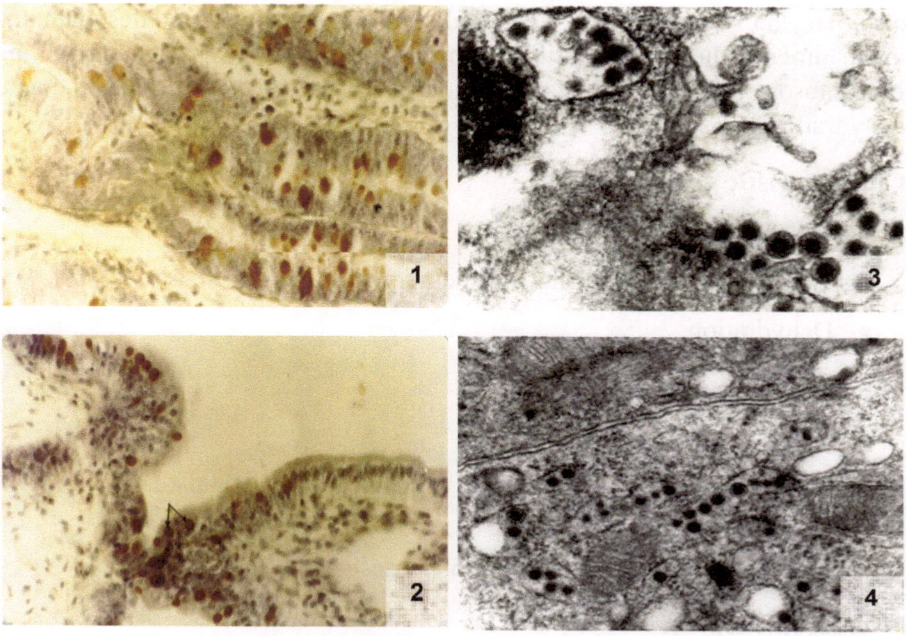

Fig. 1.15: Diagnosis of rotavirus infection in calves- Immunoperoxidase technique for demonstration of (1) Rotavirus antigen,(2) Rotavirus producing cells, (3) Transmission electronmicroscopy of the intestinal tissue showing assembly of virions and (4) Their migration through endoplasmic reticulum trabeculae.

Etiology

- Rotavirus belonging to family Reoviridae
- Double stranded RNA
- 11 segments in genome

Pathogenesis

The disease spreads either through direct contact or through contaminated water, milk and fomites. The virus infects mature epithelial cells of the small intestine due to presence of receptors in the form of beta-galactosidase on the brush border of the epithelium or the receptors of immunoglobulins (IgG) are utilized by the virus. Only differentiated columnar epithelial cell lining of apical half of villi are susceptible. The virus does not enter and replicate in immature/ proliferating cells in crypts because these cells lack receptors for the virus. Epithelial cells develop cisternae (wide spaces) in endoplasmic reticulum with swollen mitochondria. The viral particles appear in distended cisternae and lysosomes. The epithelial cells are vacuolated and desquamated in the lumen of the intestine. Villi thus become atrophic and shortened resulting in malabsorption and maldigestion. The death of affected calves occurs due to dehydration.

Characteristic symptoms

- Fever (104-106°F)
- Watery yellowish diarrhoea, dysentery with melena
- Dehydration

Macroscopic features

- Congestion of intestines
- Presence of desquamated cells mixed catarrhal exudate in the small intestines
- Enlargement of mesenteric lymph nodes

Microscopic features

- Increased number of goblet cells in villi
- Shortening of the length of villi
- Fusion of two adjacent villi
- Infiltration of mononuclear cells in mucosa and submucosa
- Congestion and hemorrhage

Diagnosis

- Symptoms and lesions
- Immunodiagnostic tests for demonstration of antigen /antibody
- AGPT
- CIEP
- ELISA
- Isolation of virus
- Demonstration of virus antigen in intestinal tissue sections using immunoperoxidase technique.

Coronavirus Infection

Coronavirus infection causes acute gastroenteritis in neonates of animal characterized by damage in villi as well as crypts leading to mal digestion, mal absorption, shortening of villi, hemorrhage in small and large intestines (Fig.1.16).

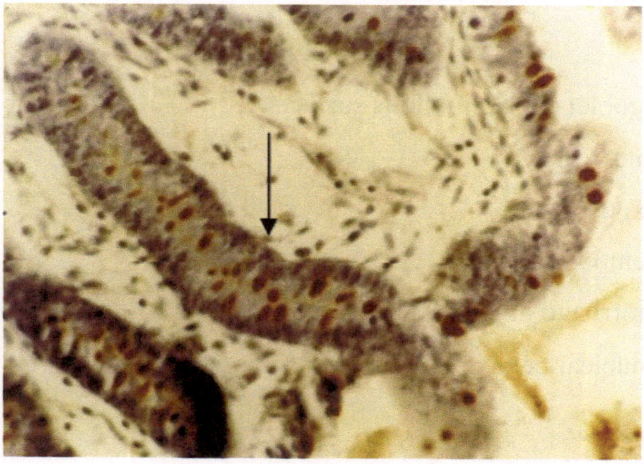

Fig. 1.16: Coronavirus infection in calves- Presence of coronovirus antigen in crypts of small intestine using immunofacroxidase technique.

Etiology

- Coronavirus

Pathogenesis

The disease spreads either through direct contact or through contaminated water, milk and fomites. The virus infects both mature and immature epithelial cells of the small intestine. Epithelial cells of crypts and villi develop cisternae (wide spaces) in endoplasmic reticulum with swollen mitochondria. The viral particles appear in distended cisternae and lysosomes. The epithelial cells are vacuolated and desquamated in the lumen of the intestine. Villi thus become atrophic and shortened resulting in malabsorption and maldigestion. The death of affected calves occurs due to dehydration and loss of blood.

Characteristic symptoms

- Fever (104-106°F)
- Diarrhoea, dysentery with melena
- Dehydration

Macroscopic features

- Congestion of small and large intestines
- Presence of muco-hemorrhagic exudate along with desquamated cells in intestine
- Enlargement of mesenteric lymph nodes

Microscopic features

- Increase number of goblet cells on villous surface
- Shortening of villi and crypts
- Hemorrhage from exposed villi
- Fusion of two adjacent villi
- Congestion and hemorrhage in mucosa and submucosa
- Infiltration of mononuclear cells in mucosa and submucosa

Diagnosis

- Symptoms and lesions
- Immunodiagnostic tests for demonstration of antigen /antibody
- CFT
- ELISA
- Isolation of virus
- Demonstration of virus antigen in intestinal tissue sections using immunoperoxidase technique

Parainfluenza-3 Infection

Parainfluenza-3 virus causes respiratory disease in cattle, sheep and goat characterized by rhinitis and bronchopneumonia

Etiology

- Parainfluenza-3 virus
- Secondary invaders
- Corynebacterium
- Streptococci
- *Pasturella multocida*

Pathogenesis

It is one of the important pathogenesis of both animal and man. Infection occurs through the respiratory route and virus multiplies in respiratory epithelium resulting in viraemia with short courses of fever, rhinitis and nasal discharge, lacrimation, coughing and dyspnoea.

Characteristic symptoms

- Fever(105-107°F)
- Nasal discharge
- Sneezing, coughing

Macroscopic features

- Congestion of nasal mucosa
- Mucopurulent exudate in upper respiratory tract
- Congestion and consolidation of lungs
- Congestion of mediastinal lymph nodes
- Lobular distribution of lesions in lungs

Microscopic features

- Infiltration of mononuclear cells in alveoli around the bronchi
- Proliferation of septal cells present in inter alveolar spaces
- Presence of giant cells in alveoli
- Presence of intra cytoplasmic and intra nuclear eosinophilic inclusions

Diagnosis

- Symptoms and lesions
- Immunodiagnostic tests for demonstration of antigen /antibody
- AGPT
- ELISA
- Isolation of virus
- Demonstration of viral antigen in respiratory tract epithelium using immunoperoxidase technique.

Bovine Immunodeficiency

Bovine immunodeficiency is an infectious viral diseases of cattle caused by lentivirus and characterized by lethargyness, abscess formation, abomasitis, lymphosarcoma and immunosuppression.

Etiology

- Lentivirus of retroviridae family
- RNA virus having reverse transcriptase enzyme

Pathogenesis

The virus mainly spreads through insect bites; though the possibility of vertical transmission cannot be ruled out. The virus replicates in macrophages and lymphocytes and remains cell associated as infection is life long leading to lymphocytolysis and immunosuppression.

Characteristic symptoms

- Lethargyness
- Abscess formation
- Mastitis, dermatitis, pneumonia or digestive disorders as a result of immunosuppression.

Macroscopic features

- Subcutaneous nodules of lymphoid follicles
- Abscess on skin
- Pododermatitis
- Lymphadenopathy

Microscopic features

- Lymphosarcoma
- Lymphocytosis or lymphopenia
- Lymphocytic encephalitis and meningitis

Diagnosis

- Symptoms and lesions
- Detection of virus antigen/antibody using ELISA

- Demonstration of viral antigen in lymphocytes using immunoperoxidase technique
- Demonstration of virus using electronmicroscopy.

Bovine Leukemia

Bovine leukemia is an infectious viral disease of cattle caused by oncornavirus characterized by malignant lymphoma in lymph nodes, lymphocytosis with immature lymphocytes in blood. It is also known as bovine lymphoma or malignant lymphoma (Fig.1.17).

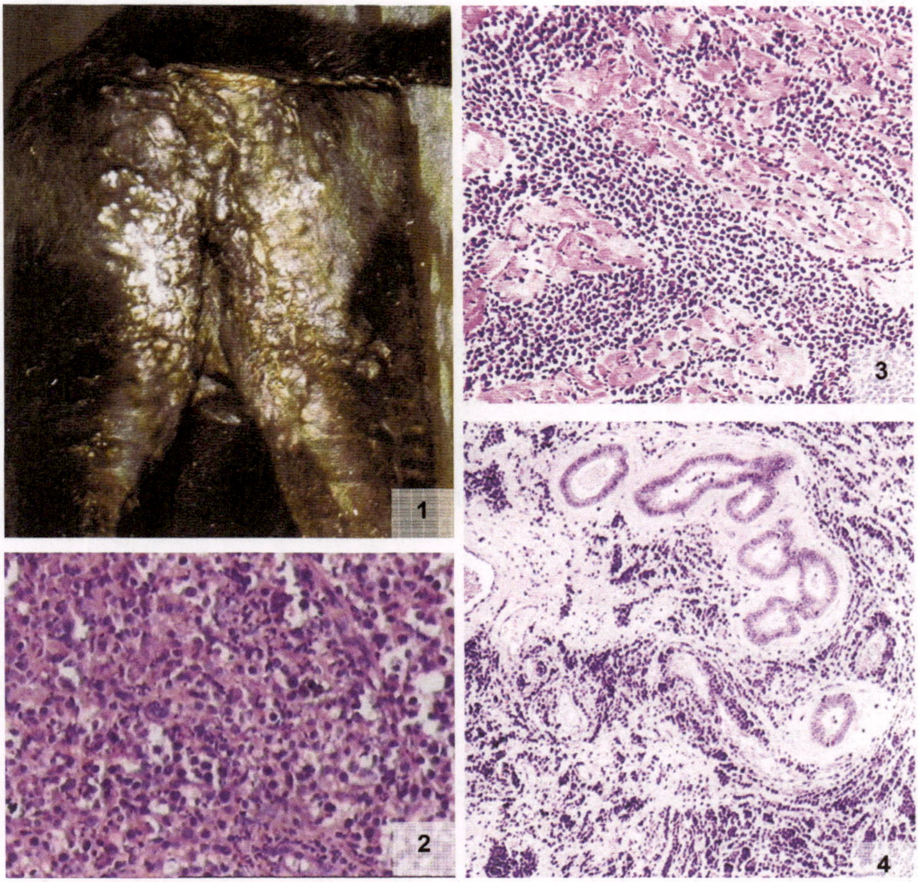

Fig. 1.17: Bovine leukemia (1) lymphoma on skin and (2,3 & 4) Microscopic features of lymphosarcoma

Etiology

- Oncorna virus of retroviridae family
- Type C oncorna virus having reverse transcriptase, RNA virus

Pathogenesis

The virus is transmitted horizontally and infects lymphocytes leading to their proliferation. The proviral DNA of virus incorporated in host cell DNA inducing neoplastic growth of the cells.

Characteristic symptoms

- Lymphocytosis
- Enlargement of superficial lymph nodes
- Weakness, emaciation, cachexia

Macroscopic features

- Enlargement of lymph nodes (mesenteric, pelvic and sublumbar)
- Dehydrated, emaciated and cachectic carcass

Microscopic features

- Immature lymphocytes in blood
- Mitotic figures, anaplastic cells in lymph nodes
- Heavy lymphocytic infiltration in myocardium

Diagnosis

- Symptoms and lesions
- Detection of antigen/antibody using ELISA
- Demonstration of viral antigen in affected tissue using IFT or immunoperoxidase technique
- Demonstration of virus using electronmicroscopy

Ephemeral Fever

Ephemeral fever is a viral disease of animals characterized by three days sickness, oedematous lymph nodes, hydropericardium, hydrothorax, pulmonary emphysema, tendovaginitis, and congestion of abomasal folds and focal necrosis of muscle.

Etiology

- Vesiculovirus of Rhabdoviridae family
- Bullet shaped RNA virus

Pathogenesis

The virus is transmissible through insects and after an incubation period of 2-10 days, viraemia sets in. Thereafter, virus localizes in the joints, lymphocytes and muscles.

Clinical Symptoms

- Three day sickness
- Shifting lameness
- High fever which subsides after 3 days
- Stiffness of joints

Macroscopic features

- Hydrothorax, hydropericardium
- Odematous lymph nodes
- Rhinitis, tracheitis, pulmonary emphysema
- Congestion of abomasum

Microscopic features

- Vascular enlargement/congestion
- Emphysema in lungs
- Focal necrosis of muscle
- Petechiae in peripheral nerves

Diagnosis

- Symptoms and lesions
- Detection of antigen and antibody using ELISA
- Demonstration of viral antigen in affected tissues using immunoperoxidase technique.

Blue Tongue

Blue tongue is an infectious viral disease of sheep caused by orbivirus and characterized by oedema and congestion of face, congestion and cyanosis of tongue, endothelial hyperplasia and arteritis (Fig.1.18).

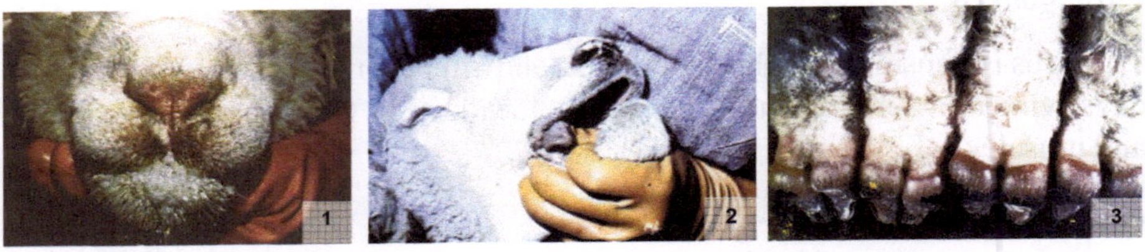

Fig. 1.18: 1. Oedema of Face, **2.** Oedema and cyanosis of tongue, **3.** Haemorrhage on coronets leading to pododermatitis

Etiology

- Orbivirus of Reoviridae family
- dsRNA virus

Pathogenesis

Blue tongue is transmitted by biting of insects including culicoids and other mosquitoes and ectoparasites like *Malophagus ovinus*. The infection has also been transmitted by insemination from an infected male, since virus is present in the semen. After infection, viral replication starts in haemopoietic cells which results in viraemia and subsequent replication in endothelial cells of blood vessels throughout the body. The damage of endothelial cells leads to development of hyperemia, hemorrhage, edema and thrombosis.

Characteristic symptoms

- Fever(105-107^{0}F)
- Oedema of face
- Cyanosis of tongue
- Signs of mosquito bite on skin

Macroscopic features

- Oedema and congestion of face, head, neck
- Oedema and cyanosis of tongue
- Petechial hemorrhage on oral and nasal mucosa

- Hemorrhage on coronets leading to pododermatitis
- Hemorrhage in abomasum and intestines.

Microscopic features

- Hemorrhage and infiltration of mononuclear cells in tongue
- Hyperemia of vascular corium of skin in coronets
- Hemorrhage in muscles of coronets
- Hemorrhage and infiltration of neutrophils in abomasum and intestines.

Diagnosis

- Symptoms and lesions
- Immunodiagnostic tests for demonstration of antigen /antibody
- AGPT
- CIEP
- ELISA
- Isolation of virus

Contagious Ecthyma

Contagious ecthyma is a highly infectious viral disease of sheep and goats characterized by the presence of pustular and scabby lesions on muzzle and lips (Fig.1.19).

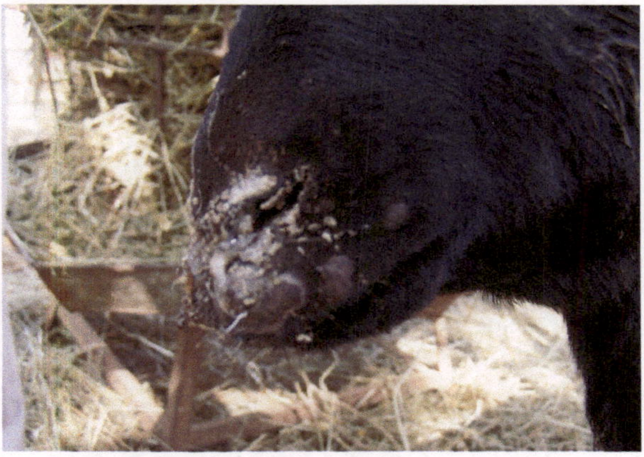

Fig. 1.19: Contagious ecthyma in goat

Etiology

- Contagious ecthyma virus belongs to poxviridae family
- Similar to pseudo-cow pox virus
- Very resistant virus

Pathogenesis

Virus transmitted through direct and indirect contact with contaminated materials like feed, fences, manure, bedding. Infected lambs may transmit the virus through suckling on teats and udder of dam. Lesions develop on mouth as papule and then pustules. These are covered with thick tenacious scabs covering a raised area of ulceration.

Characteristic symptoms

- Pustular and scabby lesions on muzzle, nostrils and lips
- Pustular lesions on coronets, ears, anus, vulva, perpura
- Morbidity is high, mortality low

Macroscopic features

- Pustular lesions on muzzle, lips and nostrils
- Gastroenteritis
- Bronchopneumonia
- Ulcers in nasal mucosa, oesophagus, abomasum and small intestines.

Microscopic features

-

Diagnosis

- Symptoms and lesions
- Immunodiagnossis- ELISA
- Demonstration of antigen in tissue sections using immunoperoxidase techniques

Pulmonary Adenomatosis

Pulmonary adenomatosis or Jaagsiekte is an infectious viral disease of sheep caused by a lentivirus and characterized by metaplasia of alveolar epithelium to cuboidal or columnar giving it an appearance of gland (Fig.1.20).

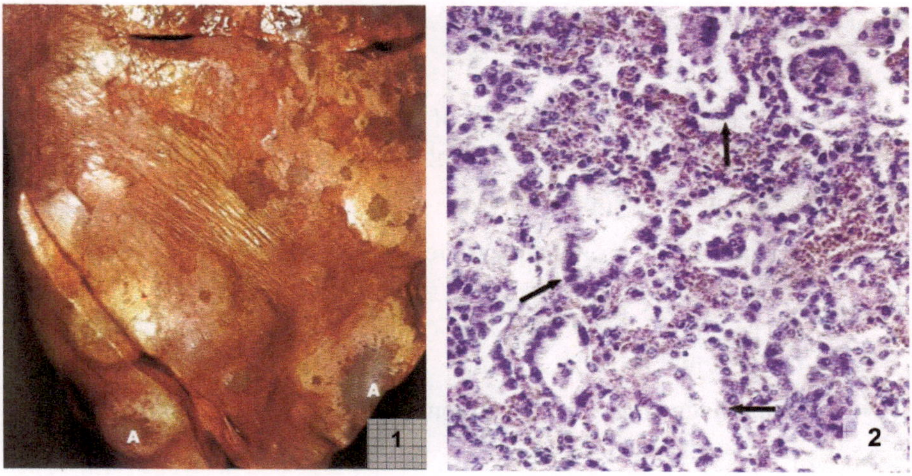

Fig. 1.20: Pulmonary adenomatosis (1) Nodules in lung (2) Metaplasia of alveolar epithelium to cuboidal (arrow).

Etiology

- Lentivirus of Retroviridae family
- RNA virus, having reverse transcriptase enzyme

Pathogenesis

It has a very long incubation period (1-3 years). It is transmitted through direct contact or droplet infection for a long period of time. The disease may also be vertically transmitted from mother to lambs. After entry virus multiplies and localizes in lungs. There is development of oedematous growth in the alveolar epithelium due to metaplasia. As a result there is interference of oxygen exchange resulting to hypoxia and anoxia.

Characteristic symptoms

- Chronic nasal discharge
- Weakness, wasting

Macroscopic features

- Nodular foci in lungs
- Congestion and consolidation of lungs
- Later stages characterized by fibrosis.

Microscopic features

- Lymphoid follicles in lungs
- Proliferation and hypertrophy of alveolar epithelial cells leading to cuboidal or columnar epithelium giving it a shape of gland
- Thickening of alveolar wall
- Adenomatosis in bronchial and mediastinal lymph nodes.

Diagnosis

- Symptoms and lesions
- Immunodiagnostic tests for demonstration of antigen /antibody
- ELISA
- Demonstration of viral antigen in lung tissues using IFT or immunoperoxidase technique.

Maedi / Visna

Maedi is an infectious chronic viral disease of sheep caused by lentivirus and characterized by encephalomyelitis and pneumonia.

Etiology

- Lentivirus of Retroviridae family
- RNA virus having reverse transcriptase enzyme

Pathogenesis

The disease is mainly transmitted through respiratory route. Mononuclear cells of infected sheep contain virus including mononuclear cells of colostrum and milk through which lambs get infected. The virus replicates in the macrophages which leads to cell associated viraemia and dissemination of the virus to the brain and other organs. The virus can not be trapped by antibodies. Antibodies are produced very slowly as a result; these antibodies are insufficient in selecting antigenically different virions. So the virus can spread between cells much faster than it can be neutralized by antibodies.

Characteristic symptoms

- Chronic nasal discharge
- Wasting

- Aimless movements

Macroscopic features

- Lungs have dense and rubbery consistency
- Lungs enlarged 2-5 times
- Cut surface is dry with no exudate
- Congestion of meninges and brain
- Enlargement of mediastinal lymph nodes, adhesive pleuritis.

Microscopic features

- Zones of demyelination with destruction of para ventricular white matter in cerebellum and cerebrum
- Gliosis and lymphocytic infiltration in brain and meninges
- Thickening of the alveolar wall due to proliferation of mononuclear cells and fibroblasts
- Alveolar lining cells become swollen and becomes cuboidal in shape.
- Intra cytoplasmic inclusions in macrophages.

Diagnosis

- Symptoms and lesions
- Immunodiagnostic tests for demonstration of antigen /antibody
- ELISA
- Demonstration of viral antigen in macrophages and/or lung tissue using immunoperoxidase technique.

Peste de Petits in Ruminants (PPR)

Peste de Petits ruminants (PPR) is an infectious viral disease of small ruminants caused by morbilli virus and characterized by giant cell pneumonia, erosive stomatitis and enteritis (Fig.1.21).

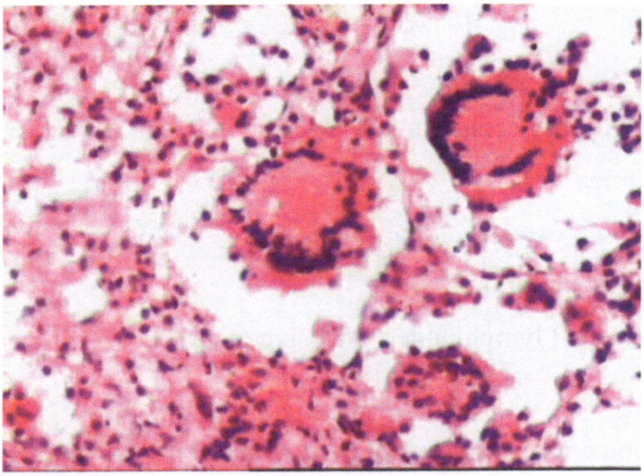

Fig. 1.21: PPR in sheep and goats A. Nasal discharge, B. Erosive mouth lesions and hemorrhage at gum-teeth junctions, C. Blood mixed diarrhea, D. Linea hemorrhage (Zebra markings) and E. Giant cell pneumonia.

Etiology

- Morbilli virus of Paramyxoviridae family
- RNA virus, very frazile virus

Pathogenesis

Infection is mainly transmitted by inhalation through close contact with infected animals. After entry virus penetrate retropharyngeal lymph nodes and mucosa and multiplies there that leads to viraemia. The virus reaches mucous membrane of alimentary and respiratory tract where it proliferates and causes damage to them. There is inflammation of mucosa leading to enteritis, diarrhoea, dehydration and death in young animals. Due to inflammation of lungs, giant cell pneumonia and respiratory distress develops. In PPR, lymphoid necrosis is not high as in rinderpest. Most of sheep and some adult goats recover and they carry antibodies that provide life long immunity.

Characteristic symptoms

- Fever (105-107°C)
- Diarrhoea, melena
- Erosive mouth lesions
- Skin eruptions

- Conjunctivitis
- Mortality up to 80%

Macroscopic features

- Congestion and consolidation of lungs
- Hemorrhagic / erosive enteritis
- Erosive mouth lesions
- Erosive lesions in large intestine in strips along payers patches giving rise to ***"Zebra markings"*** in large intestine

Microscopic features

- Giant cell pneumonia
- Erosions in oral mucous membrane
- Erosions in intestinal mucous membrane
- Hemorrhage and congestion in intestines
- Infiltration of mononuclear cells
- Depletion of lymphoid cells in lymph nodes.

Diagnosis

- Symptoms and lesions
- Immunodiagnostic tests for demonstration of antigen /antibody
- AGPT
- CIEP
- ELISA
- Isolation of virus
- Demonstration of viral antigen in lung and intestinal tissue using immunoperoxidase technique.

Swine Fever (Hog Cholera)

Swine fever is an acute contagious viral disease of pigs caused by pestivirus of Togaviridae family and characterized by gluing of eyes, congestion and widespread haemorrhage in visceral organs (Fig.1.22).

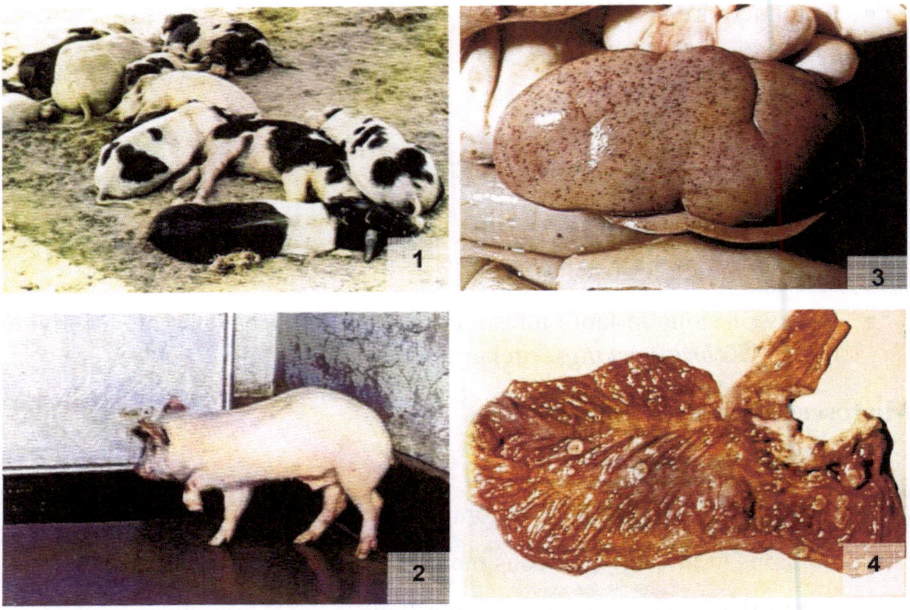

Fig. 1.22: Swine fever (hog cholera)- (1) Hurdling of big lets (2) Goose stepping, (3) Petechia on kidney and (4) Button ulcers in intestines.

Etiology

- Pestivirus of Togaviridae family
- RNA virus

Pathogenesis

Pig is the only domestic animal which is naturally infected by the virus. Infection is usually acquired by ingestion but inhalation is also a possible route. The source of virus is always infected pig and its products. In infected pig, virus is found in all excretions and secretions of body. After ingestion, virus reaches in the tonsils, where primary multiplication of virus occurs within few hours of infection. Then virus is transported through lymphatics and enter in blood capillaries resulting in an initial viraemia by about 24 hours of infection. As time goes on, virus spreads to different tissues like spleen, peripheral and visceral lymph nodes, bone marrow, Peyer's patches. The virus causes destruction of endothelial cells, lymphoreticular cells, macrophages and epithelial cells. Virus causes hydropic degeneration and proliferation of vascular endothelium which results in occlusion of blood vessels leading to congestion, hemorrhage and infarction in arterioles, venules and capillaries. In small and medium sized arteries, thrombosis is also seen. At early stages, there is leucopenia followed by leucocytosis.

Characteristic symptoms

- Fever(105-106°F)
- Gluing of eyes
- Herd ling
- Congestion of skin with eruptions
- Mortality up to 100%

Macroscopic features

- Gluing of eyes
- Congestion and hemorrhage in kidneys, lymph nodes, urinary bladder, skin, spleen, lungs and large intestines
- Button ulcers in large intestines
- Erythema and cyanosis on ventral abdomen and thorax skin.

Microscopic features

- Perivascular cuffing in brain by lymphocytes, monocytes and plasma cells
- Intranuclear, round, homogenous acidophilic inclusion in neurons
- Hemorrhage in spleen, lymph nodes and kidneys
- Necrosis of mucosa and submucosa in intestines leading to formation of ulcers and infiltration of mononuclear cells.

Diagnosis

- Symptoms and lesions
- Immunodiagnostic tests for demonstration of antigen /antibody
- AGPT
- CIEP
- ELISA
- Demonstration of viral antigen in affected tissues using immunoperoxidase technique.
- Isolation of virus

Transmissible Gastroenteritis

Transmissible gastroenteritis is contagious viral disease of pigs caused by corona virus and characterized by vomiting, diarrhoea, dehydration with high mortality.

Etiology

- Corona virus
- RNA virus

Pathogenesis

Transmission of virus occurs through inhalation and ingestion. Virus infects mature enterocytes of intestinal villi causing their necrosis and desquamation leading to atrophy of villi.

Characteristic symptoms

- Diarrhoea
- Vomiting
- Dehydration
- Morbidity and mortality 100%

Macroscopic features

- Dehydrated carcass
- Curdled milk in stomach
- Congestion of small intestine
- Petechiae in intestines

Microscopic features

- Shortening and fusion of villi, villous atrophy
- Cuboidal epithelium on villous surface
- Absence of microvilli, vacuolation in epithelial cells
- Infiltration of mononuclear cells in mucosa and submucosa

Diagnosis

- Symptoms and lesions

- Detection of viral antigen in faeces or antibody in serum using ELISA
- Demonstration of viral antigen in enterocytes using immunoperoxidase technique
- Demonstration of virus using by electronmicroscopy

Pseudorabies

Pseudorabies is a viral disease of animals, mainly of swine and characterized by itching, in coordination, tremors, convulsions, paralysis and encephalitis.

Etiology

- Herpes virus- *Herpes suis*
- DNA virus

Pathogenesis

After intranasal or entry through skin, the virus takes 7-8 days to localize in peripheral nerves. Where it causes necrosis of muscles and fascia and travels to spinal cord and brain to cause encephalomyelitis.

Clinical Symptoms

- Fever, itching
- In coordination of hind limbs
- Tremors, paralysis, convulsions
- Scratching due to itching
- Respiratory failure leads to death

Macroscopic features

- Encephalitis
- Scratch wounds due to itching
- Enlargement of lymph nodes

Microscopic features

- Necrosis of nerve fibers and ganglion
- Lymphocytic infiltration
- Intra nuclear inclusion in nerve cells, ganglion and schwann cells

- Focal necrosis of pharyngeal mucosa, tonsils, lymph nodes, lungs and liver

Diagnosis

- Symptoms and lesions
- Detection of antigen and/or antibody using ELISA
- Demonstration of viral antigen in affected tissues using immunoperoxidase technique.

Equine Influenza

Equine influenza is contagious viral diseases of horses caused by orthomyxovirus and characterized by fever, coughing and pandemic occurrence of the disease.

Etiology

- Influenza A virus of orthomyxoviridae family
- Very unstable virus, frequent antigenic drift and shift

Pathogenesis

Virus spreads through inhalation and multiplies in respiratory epithelium causing erythema, oedema and focal erosions. There is very mild and short viremia.

Characteristic symptoms

- Fever (101 – 106°F)
- Coughing
- Nasal discharge
- Oedema and pain in superficial lymph nodes

Macroscopic features

- Erosions in upper respiratory mucosa
- Peribronchitis, bronchitis
- Bronchopneumonia

Microscopic features

- Hyaline membrane formation on bronchiolar and alveolar epithelium
- Peribronchitis, bronchitis and bronchopneumonia

Diagnosis

- Symptoms and lesions
- Detection of antigen / antibody using haemagglutination, haemagglutination inhibition test, ELISA
- Demonstration of viral antigen in affected tissue using immunoperoxidase technique
- Demonstration of virus in tissue/secretions using electronmicroscopy

Equine Infectious Anemia

Equine infectious anemia is a viral disease of horses caused by lentivirus and characterized by icterus, anemia, hyperemia and oedema of sub cutis of the ventral wall of abdomen, pleura, heart, spleen and lymph nodes.

Etiology

- Lentivirus of Retroviridae family
- RNA virus having reverse transcriptase enzyme

Pathogenesis

The disease is transmitted mechanically by the bite of mosquito (Culex) or biting flies (Stomoxys, Tebanus). It can also be transmitted by unsterilized needles, comb, saddle,etc. through minute transfer of blood from infected animal. After entry virus multiples in various organs like spleen, kidneys, lymph nodes and liver. After 30 days of viraemia virus attacks erythrocytes and cause their destruction. It also causes destruction of endothelial cells of blood vessels, peripheral nerves, meninges, and brain tissue leading to the development of nervous signs. The hemolytic anemia develops due to hemolysis and phagocytosis of erythrocytes by reticuloendothelial system. Virus antibody complex may be deposited on the renal glomerulus causing glomerulonephritis.

Characteristic symptoms

- Anemia
- Icterus
- Chronic wasting/ weakness
- Oedema of dependent parts of body

Macroscopic features

- Oedema in ventral abdomen
- Petechial or ecchymotic haemorrhage on pleura, peritoneum and serosa of visceral organs
- Enlargement of spleen, liver and lymph nodes
- Increased red marrow in bones specially in long bones.

Microscopic features

- Congestion, haemorrhage and oedema in visceral organs
- Infiltration of immature lymphoid cells in liver, kidneys, heart etc.
- Erythro-phagocytosis in spleen
- Dilatation of sinusoids due to congestion and filled with lymphoid cells.

Diagnosis

- Symptoms and lesions
- Immunodiagnostic tests for demonstration of antigen /antibody
- ELISA
- Demonstration of viral antigen in affect tissues using immunoperoxidase technique.

Equine Encephalomyelitis

Equine encephalomyelitis is an arboviral disease characterized by circling movements, high fever, paralysis, neuronophagia and perivascular cuffing. This is also known as ***staggers, borna disease*** or ***forage poisoning***.

Etiology

- Group A arbovirus of alphavirus
- Western, eastern and Venezuelan strains

Pathogenesis

The virus spreads through mosquitoes and birds, reptiles and rodents are the resinous of the virus. With an incubation period of 10-15 days, clinical signs of fever and aimless walking appear in horse.

Clinical Symptoms

- Aimless walking, circling movements
- Fever
- Paralysis

Macroscopic features

- No characteristics gross lesions
- Congestion of meninges and brain

Microscopic features

- Encephalomalacia
- Neuronophagia, chromatolysis
- Perivascular cuffing by lymphocytes
- Intra nuclear acidophilic inclusion bodies in neurons

Diagnosis

- Symptoms, lesions
- Detection of antigen or antibody using ELISA
- Demonstration of viral antigen in nerve cells using immunoperoxidase technique.

Equine Viral Arteritis

Equine viral arteritis is an infectious disease of horse, mules and donkeys characterized by palpebral oedema, abortion, enteritis and pneumonia.

Etiology

- Pestivirus of Togaviridae family
- RNA virus 40-70 nm diameter

Pathogenesis

Virus reaches in body through inhalation and viraemia occurs causing severe damage to small arteries in intestines, lymph nodes and adrenals that leads to diarrhoea and abdominal pain. It causes severe myometritis, conjunctivitis and pulmonary oedema.

Clinical Symptoms

- Oedema in limbs
- Conjunctivitis
- Abortion
- Diarrhoea
- Panleucopenia

Macroscopic features

- Enteritis
- Palpebral oedema
- Pneumonia, enlargement of mediastinal lymph nodes
- Placentitis
- Hydrothorax

Microscopic features

- Widespread oedema in lungs placenta with congestion and haemorrhage.
- Arteritis in caecum and colon-characterized by deposition of eosinophilic material in media with cellular infiltration

Diagnosis

- Symptoms and lesions
- Detection of antigen and antibody using ELISA
- Demonstration of viral antigen in affected tissues using immunoperoxidase technique.

African Horse Sickness

African horse sickness is an acute viral disease of horses caused by orbivirus and characterized by fever, conjunctivitis, and oedema of lungs, heart and neck. This is also known as ***equine plague***.

Etiology

- Orbivirus of reoviridae family
- dsRNA with 10 segments

Pathogenesis

Virus enters in body through inhalation and after an incubation period of 7-10 days, it causes oedema in lungs with laboured breathing. There is several liters of water accumulates in thorax.

Clinical Symptoms

- Fever
- Dyspnoea
- Coughing
- Foamy discharges from nostrils

Macroscopic features

- Hydrothorax
- Pulmonary oedema
- Sub endocardial haemorrhage
- Conjunctivitis

Microscopic features

- Pulmonary oedema characterized by separation of interlobular tissue from alveoli
- Infiltration of mononuclear cells in inter alveolar spaces
- Sub endocardial haemorrhage
- Necrosis in liver

Diagnosis

- Symptoms and lesions
- Demonstration of antibody or antigen using ELISA
- Demonstration of viral antigen in affected tissues using immunoperoxidase technique.

Equine Viral Abortion (EHV infection)

Equine viral abortion is caused by herpes virus and characterized by death of foetus, abortion, retained placenta and post parturient metritis.

Etiology

- Equine herpes virus-1 of herpesviridae family
- DNA virus

Pathogenesis

The virus spreads through inhalation or ingestion of contaminated material. On entry, virus affects the macrophages and remains in latency till suitable conditions. It affects the placenta, foetus causing placentitis and death of foetus near completion of gestation that results in abortion.

Characteristic symptoms

- Abortion in late gestation
- Retained placenta
- Vaginal discharges

Macroscopic features

- Necrotic lesions on lung, liver and lymph nodes of aborted foetus
- Metritis
- Placentitis

Microscopic features

- Necrosis in liver of aborted foetus
- Intra nuclear eosinophilic inclusion bodies in hepatocytes, spleen, lymph nodes and bronchioles
- Interlobular oedema in lungs
- Bronchopneumonia

Diagnosis

- Symptoms and lesions
- Detection of viral antigen/antibody using ELISA
- Demonstration of viral antigen in affected tissue by immunoperoxidase technique
- Demonstration of virus using electronmicroscopy

Equine rhinopneumonitis

Equine rhinopneumonitis is a contagions viral disease of foals caused by EHV-1 & 4 and characterized by respiratory distress, pneumonia and death.

Etiology

- Equine herpes virus (EHV-1 and EHV-4).
- DNA virus.

Pathogenesis

- Transmission – aerosol, inhalation through virus laden respiratory secretions / discharges.
- Viremia, localizes in respiratory system.
- Rhinopneumonitis.

Clinical Manifestations

- Fever, nasal discharge, coughing, sneezing.
- Death occurs due to asphyxia.

Macroscopic features

- Pneumonia
- Congestion & hemorrhage in trachea.
- Plugging in bronchi.
- Encephalopathy.

Microscopic features

- Bronchopneumonia.
- Hyaline membrane over bronchial and alveolar epithelium.
- Tracheitis, bronchitis.
- Meningoencephatitis.

Diagnosis

- Symptoms and lesions
- Agent identification – Serology, PCR.

Rabies

Rabies is a viral disease of animals mainly affecting carnivores like dogs, wolves, foxes caused by a lyssa virus and characterized by encephalitis, and presence of intra cytoplasmic inclusions in nerve cells (Fig.1.23).

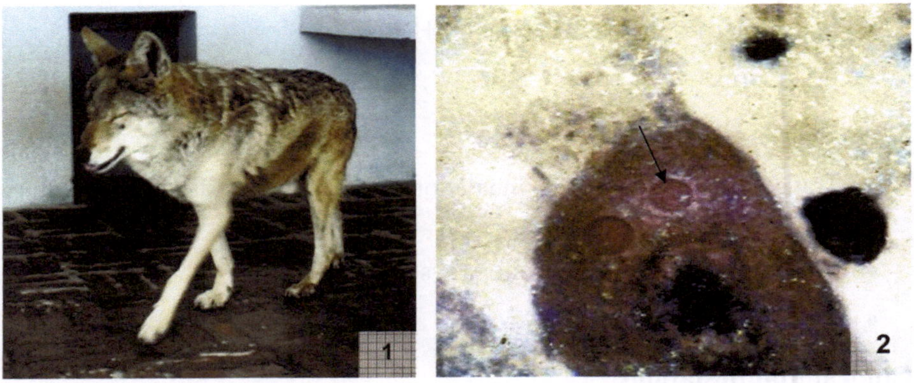

Fig. 1.23: Rabies (1) Dumb form in a wolf (2) Intracytoplasmic eosinophilic inclusion body (Negri body) (arrow).

Etiology

- Lyssa virus of Rhabdoviridae family
- Bullet shaped, RNA virus

Pathogenesis

The source of infection is always an infected animal and method of spread is almost always by bite of a rabid animal. The virus may appear in the milk of affected animals but spread through this means remains doubtful. After entry of the virus, there is incubation period of 1 week to 1 year with a mean of 1-2 months. Several factors play role in establishing rabies include virulence of the strain, quantity of infectious virus in saliva and susceptibility of the species. Length of incubation period depends on anatomical distance between bite site and the central nervous system, severity of the bite and amount of infectious virus in the saliva.

After entry virus first replicates in the muscle cells and sheds into extra-cellular spaces. Then virus enters into nervous system at motor end plates and binds to receptors for acetylcholine (Ach). After reaching peripheral/ central nerves, the virus spreads within axon of nerve cells to the ventral horn cells of spinal cord @ 3-4 mm/hour. Virus multiplication occurs first in the spinal cord and then spreads to the brain and from where it is disseminated throughout the central nervous system. During dissemination to central nervous system, there is no viraemia. Direct trans neural transfer of virus from cell bodies of neurons and dendrites to adjacent axon terminals is a mechanism of dissemination of rabies in the central nervous system. Brain stem, cerebral cortex and hippocampus are mainly affected by rabies virus and destruction of these regions gives rise to clinical symptoms of rabies. There is centrifugal spread via nerves throughout the body including salivary gland, cornea and tonsils. The virus replicates rapidly in salivary gland and such saliva is the major source of infection for susceptible animals. When there is irritation phenomenon (induced by virus in the nerve cells) occurs, which causes external i.e. furious form and when destruction of neurons occurs resulting in paralysis *i.e.* paralytic/ dumb form.

Characteristic symptoms

- Drooling of saliva
- Moving aimlessly
- Eating of non food materials

Macroscopic features

- No characteristic gross lesions except some wooden or non food items present in the stomach of dog.
- In other animals, lesions of bite on skin must be present

Microscopic features

- Necrosis of neurons, neuronophagic nodules, perivascular cuffing with lymphocytes in brain particularly hippocampus
- Proliferation of lymphocytes, plasma cells, glial cells replacing neurons form ***Babes nodules***
- Intra cytoplasmic eosinophilic inclusions '***Negri bodies***'

Diagnosis

- History of bite
- Symptoms and lesions
- Immunodiagnostic tests for demonstration of antigen /antibody
- IFT
- ELISA

- Isolation of virus
- Mouse inoculation test

Infectious Canine Hepatitis

Infectious canine hepatitis is an infectious viral disease of dogs caused by adenovirus characterized by necrotic lesions in liver and intra nuclear inclusions in hepatocytes.

Etiology

- Mastadenovirus of adenoviridae family
- DNA virus

Pathogenesis

The excretion of virus occurs in urine and infection spreads mainly through naso-oral and conjunctiva routes. Initial infection occurs in tonsils and peyer's patches. There is viraemia and infection of endothelial and parenchymal cells in many tissues leading to haemorrhage and necrosis, especially in the liver, kidneys, spleen and lungs. Chronic kidney lesions and corneal clouding "***blue eye***" results from immune- complex reactions.

Characteristic symptoms

- Fever(104-106°F)
- Vomiting, diarrhoea
- Icterus
- Conjunctivitis

Macroscopic features

- Enlargement and congestion of liver
- Presence of focal necrotic patches
- Thickening of the wall of gall bladder
- Enlargement of spleen
- Hyperemia of conjunctiva

Microscopic features

- Necrosis of hepatocytes leading to formation of focal necrotic foci
- Infiltration of mononuclear cells
- Intra nuclear inclusions in hepatocytes and Kupffer cells of liver, kidneys and brain
- Congestion, vascular dilatation of sinusoids

Diagnosis

- Symptoms and lesions
- Demonstration of intra nuclear inclusions in hepatocytes
- Immunodiagnostic tests for demonstration of antigen /antibody
- AGPT
- CIEP
- ELISA
- Demonstration of viral antigen in hepatocytes using immunoperoxidase technique.

Canine Distemper

Canine distemper is an infectious viral disease of dogs caused by a morbilli virus and characterized by catarrhal and purulent exudate in nasal mucosa, purulent bronchopneumonia, and vesicular/pustular dermatitis (Fig.1.24).

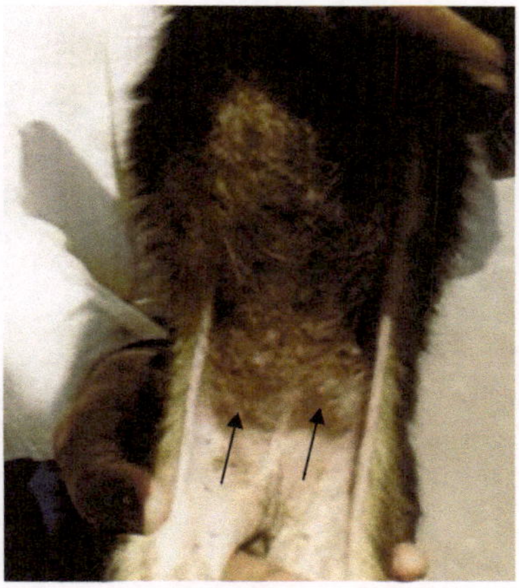

Fig. 1.24: Canine distemper- Pustules on abdomen (arrow).

Etiology

- Morbilli virus of Paramyxoviridae family
- RNA virus, very frazil virus

Pathogenesis

The route of infection is through inhalation of aerosol droplets from infected animal. After entry of virus through respiratory tract, it starts multiplication in respiratory epithelium and alveolar macrophages. Thereafter virus spreads to the tonsils and bronchial lymph nodes. Before appearance of clinical manifestations, the virus circulates in blood associated with lymphocytes and spreads to various tissue like bone marrow, spleen, brain and other lymphoid tissues. Viral replication causes direct damage to neurons and astrocytes. Indirect damage to oligodendroglial cells results in demyelination which leads to encephalitis.

In distemper encephalitis and extensive demyelination of neurons occur in chronic cases as a result of local antiviral response. The brain macrophages ingest these immune complexes and infected cells as a result they release free radicals and other toxic products. These products damage neighbouring cells especially oligodendroglia and cause demyelination. This demyelination develops as a result of autoimmune attack. In this syndrome antibodies are induced against myelin proteins which causes tissue destruction.

Characteristic symptoms

- Fever(105-107°F)
- Mucopurulent nasal discharge
- Vesicles and pustules on abdominal skin
- Foot pad becomes hard due to hyperkeratinization

Macroscopic features

- Catarrhal and purulent exudate in upper respiratory tract
- Lobular pneumonia
- Congestion and consolidation of lungs
- Hyperkeratinization of foot pad skin
- Presence of pustules on lower abdomen

Microscopic features

- Bronchopneumonia characterized by infiltration of neutrophils in alveoli around bronchioles
- Presence of intra cytoplasmic and intra nuclear eosinophilic inclusions in epithelial cells of upper respiratory passage, bronchioles, urinary bladder, stomach, skin and in circulating neutrophils

Diagnosis

- Symptoms and lesions
- Demonstration of intra nuclear and intra cytoplasmic inclusions in hepatocytes, epithelium of bronchioles, skin and in circulating neutrophils.
- Immunodiagnostic tests for demonstration of antigen /antibody
- AGPT
- CIEP
- ELISA
- Demonstration of viral antigen in hepatocytes and respiratory tract epithelium using immunoperoxidase technique.

Canine Parvoviral Infection

Parvovirus causes acute gastroenteritis in dogs characterized by necrotising enteritis and myocardial necrosis

Etiology

- Canine Parvovirus of Parvoviridae family
- DNA virus

Pathogenesis

Young dogs are mostly affected. Infection enters in body through oropharyngeal route and virus starts replication in pharyngeal lymphoid tissues. From here virus is distributed to other organs and tissues via blood stream. Cells that are in 'S' phase of cell cycle have receptors for virus and are infected and killed or prevented from entering mitosis. There is development of characteristic leucopenia involving all white blood cells-lymphocytes, neutrophils, monocytes and platelets due to their destruction.

Rapidly dividing intestinal epithelial cells in crypts are very susceptible to infection. The loss of cells from villous tips continues in normal fusion but the failure in replacing these cells with cells from crypts leads to greatly shortened, non absorptive villi and hence resulting in diarrhoea.

Characteristic symptoms

- Fever(104-106°F)
- Diarrhoea, dysentery with melena
- Dehydration

Macroscopic features

- Congestion of intestines
- Presence of mucohaemorrhagic exudate mixed with desquamated cells in lumen of intestines
- Necrosis in myocardium
- Enlargement of mesenteric lymph nodes

Microscopic features

- Necrosis of villous and crypt epithelial cells
- Dilatation of crypts
- Intra nuclear inclusions in intestinal epithelium
- Infiltration of mononuclear cells in mucosa and sub mucosa of intestines
- Myocardial necrosis surrounded by infiltration of mononuclear cells.

Diagnosis

- Symptoms and lesions
- Demonstration of intra nuclear inclusions in intestinal epithelial cells
- Immunodiagnostic tests for demonstration of antigen /antibody
- AGPT
- CIEP
- ELISA
- Demonstration of viral antigen in intestinal epithelium using immunoperoxidase technique

Feline Leukemia

Feline leukemia is an infectious viral disease of cats caused by oncorna virus and characterized by malignant lymphoma, lymphocytosis and immunosuppression. It is also known as feline lymphoma or feline lymphosarcoma.

Etiology

- Oncorna virus of retroviridae family
- Type C oncorna virus, RNA virus has reverse transcriptase

Pathogenesis

The virus is transmitted horizontally through salivary and nasal secretions of sick cats. It affects lymphocytes causing their proliferation leading to production of neoplastic growth.

Characteristic symptoms

- Enlargement of superficial lymph nodes
- Lymphocytosis
- Chronic diarrhoea
- Abortion

Macroscopic features

- Enlargement of lymph nodes (mesenteric, lumbar)
- Enteritis
- Anemia
- Placentitis

Microscopic features

- Lymphocytosis
- Anaplastic lymphoid cells in lymph nodes

Diagnosis

- Symptoms and lesions
- Detection of viral antigen/antibody using ELISA
- Demonstration of viral antigen using immunoperoxidase technique
- Demonstration of virus using electron microscopy

2

Pathology of Bacterial Diseases

Tuberculosis

Tuberculosis is a chronic bacterial disease of cattle, buffaloes, sheep, goat and pigs caused by *Mycobacterium* sp. and characterized by presence of tubercle nodules in lungs, spleen and lymph nodes (Fig.2.1).

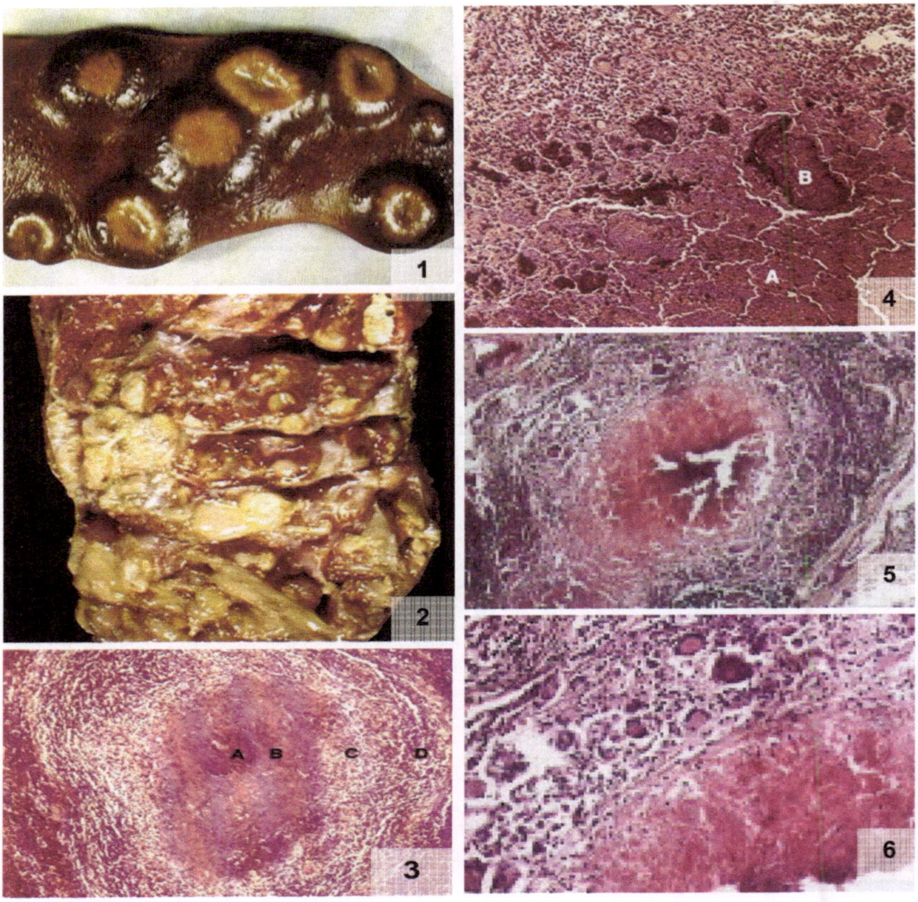

Fig. 2.1: Tuberculosis in animals- (1) Granulomatous lesions in spleen, (2) in lungs, (3) Microscopic features of tuberculosis- A. Calcification, B. Caseation, C. Macrophages and D. Fibrous covering, (4) A. Caseation and B. Calcification and giant cell (arrow), (5) Tubercle and (6) A. Giant cells, B. Caseation and C. Calcification.

Etiology

- *Mycobacterium tuberculosis*
- *M. bovis*

Pathogenesis

Disease spreads through contact with infected animals or their discharges or morbid tissues. The infected animals release the organisms through sputum at coughing and contact animals get infection through droplet inhalation.

Besides sputum, faeces, urine, vaginal discharges, semen, milk, lymph and wound discharges may act source of infection. It is also transmitted through contaminated instruments, utensils and beddings. After entry through inhalation or ingestion, bacilli localizes at the point of entry and produce typical tubercle in associated lymph nodes. Mostly pharyngeal and mesenteric lymph nodes are affected. From lymph nodes, infection may extend across body cavities, blood vessels and lymph vessels. The inhaled organism enter in the bronchial tree after lodging in bronchi a tissue reaction takes place. Neutrophilic infiltration is there and when neutrophils are necrosed, macrophages come to destroy the organism but they fail then many macrophages becomes elongated to form epithelioid cells, the hall mark of granulomatous inflammation. Some macrophages are joint together to form giant cells to destroy the acid fast bacilli. As a consequence of this some bacilli are phagocytosed and are destroyed. A zone of lymphocytes, macrophages, epithelioid cells, giant cells and fibrous connective tissues are formed around the central necrosed area.

Characteristic symptoms

- Low grade fever
- Progressive wasting/weakness, loss of production
- Coughing

Macroscopic features

- Consolidation of lungs
- Nodules of tubercle present in lungs containing cheesy mass
- Granulomatous lesions in spleen, lymph nodes, liver and intestines.
- Tubercle on pleura and mesentery (***pearly disease***).

Microscopic features

- Granulomatous lesions characterized by the presence of tubercles in different organs
- Tubercle consists of central caseative necrosed area surrounded by macrophages, lymphocytes, epithelioid cells and giant cells
- In older cases central necrosed area is calcified and surrounded by fibrous tissue capsule.

Diagnosis

- Symptoms and lesions
- Tuberculin testing of animals
- Immunodiagnostic tests for demonstration of antigen /antibody
- ELISA
- Demonstration of acid fast bacilli in impression smears of tubercle or in tissue sections of lungs and lymph nodes.

Paratuberculosis (Johne's Disease)

Paratuberculosis is a chronic bacterial disease of bovines, ovines and caprines caused by *Mycobacterium paratuberculosis* and characterized by dehydration, emaciation, chronic diarrhoea and thickening of the intestine (***corrugations***) (Fig.2.2).

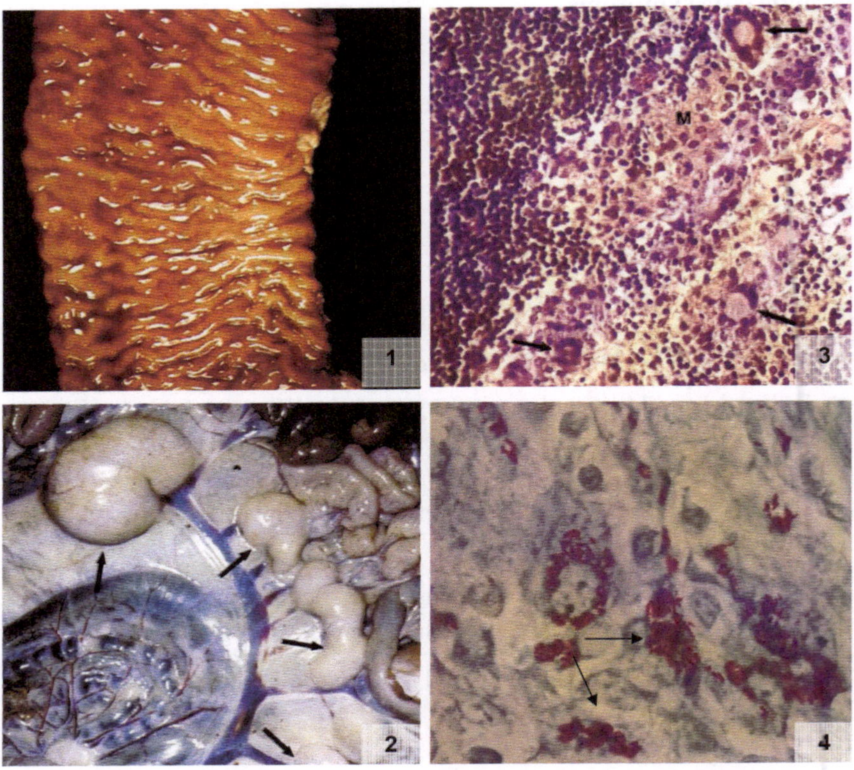

Fig. 2.2: Paratuberculosis in cattle and sheep- (1) Corrugations in large intestine, (2) Enlargement of mesenteric lymph nodes, (3) Microscopic lesions in intestine- M. Macrophages and Giant cells (arrow) and (4) Acid fast bacilli in tissue section (arrow).

Etiology

- *Mycobacterium paratuberculosis*

Pathogenesis

Faeces containing the organism is primary source of infection which is acquired by ingestion of contaminated feed and water. It has very long incubation period (15-18 months). The organism has also been isolated from genitalia and semen of infected bulls. Following infection, organism localizes in intestinal mucosa and its associated lymph nodes. The organism penetrate the intestinal mucosa and set up residence within macrophages. The organism multiplies intracellularly without killing host cells and are resistant to intracellular digestion. They grow inside macrophages and distributed through out body. The primary site for bacterial multiplication is terminal ileum and the large intestine leading to decreased absorptive surface, chronic diarrhoea and malabsorption.

Characteristic symptoms

- Chronic diarrhoea
- Progressive wasting/weakness, loss of production
- Hide bound condition

Macroscopic features

- Emaciation, cachexia
- Thickening of the intestinal wall
- Presence of '***rugae***' or transverse folds thickened due to chronic inflammatory changes
- Corrugations cannot be removed even after stretching of intestinal wall
- Lymph nodes (Mesenteric) are also enlarged.

Microscopic features

- Infiltration of macrophages, epithelioid cells and lymphocytes in mucosa and sub mucosa
- Presence of acid fast bacilli in epithelioid cells
- Absence of caseative necrosis and calcification in cattle. However, it is present in sheep and goat.
- Nests of epithelioid cells in mesenteric lymph nodes.

Diagnosis

- Symptoms and lesions
- Demonstration of acid fast bacteria in rectal pinch
- Johnin testing of animals
- Immunodiagnostic tests for demonstration of antigen /antibody
- ELISA
- Demonstration of organisms in tissue sections using special stains and immunoperoxidase technique.

Brucellosis

Brucellosis is an infectious bacterial disease of animals caused by *Brucella* sp. and characterized by abortion in late gestation and formation of granulomatous lesions in genital organs, joints and fetal liver (Fig.2.3 & Fig.2.4).

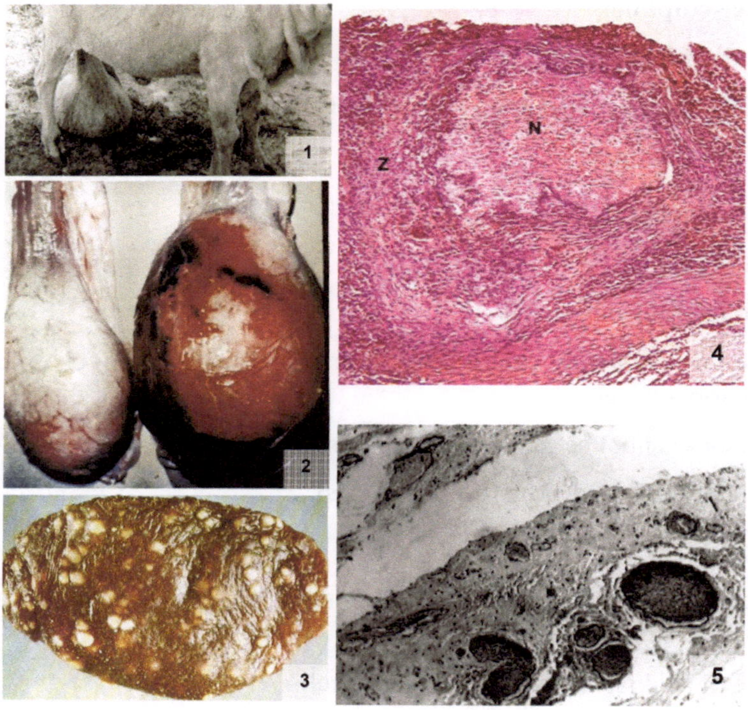

Fig. 2.3: Brucellosis in animals- (1) Orchitis in ram, (2) A. Enlargement of festicle, (3) Granulomatous lesions in spleen, (4) Microscopic features in spleen including caseation (N) and Zone of inflammatory cells (Z) and (5) Microscopic features of placenta-oedema, congestion.

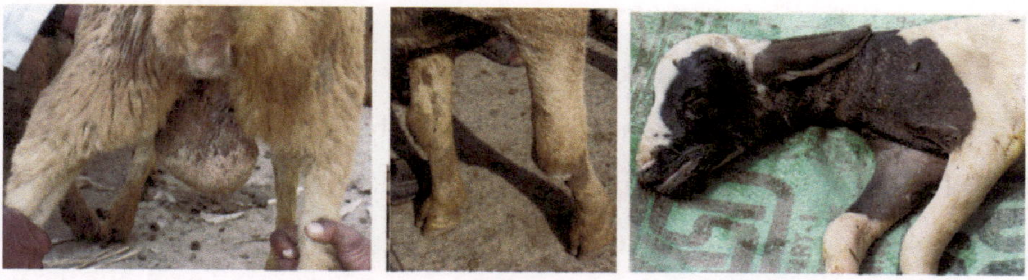

Fig. 2.4: Brucellosis in animals- A. Orchitis in ram, B. Hygroma- arthritis in sheep and aborted foetus of cattle.

Etiology

- *Brucella abortus*
- *Br. ovis*
- *Br. meletensis*
- *Br. canis*

Pathogenesis

The brucella organism spreads through ingestion of contaminated feed and water with aborted foetal contents or foetal membrane. It is also transmitted through inhalation and may pierce the intact or abraded skin or conjunctivae. Congenital infection may also occur. After entry bacteria multiply in reticuloendothelial cells in regional lymph nodes. The organism enter and travel through intestinal epithelial cells overlaying peyer's patches by endocytosis and then enters into lymphatics. The brucella organism has specific affinity with female and male reproductive organs, placenta, foetus and mammary glands. The organism can also localize in other organs like lymph nodes, spleen, liver, joints and bones. The bacteria proliferates intracellularly and it has high affinity with erythritol sugar which is present in abundance in placenta and foetus. This organism causes abortions in animals in late gestation.

Characteristic symptoms

- Orchitis
- Accumulation of fluid in scrotum
- Abortion in late gestation (7-9 month)
- Retention of placenta

Macroscopic features

- Oedema of chorion, thickened and leathery chorion/placenta
- Oedema of foetus, serosanguinous fluid in body cavity
- Pneumonia, necrotic foci in liver
- Enlargement of scrotum in males
- Induration of mammary gland in cows.

Microscopic features

- Infiltration of phagocytic cells, epithelioid cells and lymphocytes surrounded by fibrous tissue proliferation
- Fetal broncho pneumonia
- Organism in chorionic epithelial cells
- In males, proliferation of fibrous tissue which compresses or replaces the epididymis.

Diagnosis

- Symptoms and lesions
- Immunodiagnostic tests for demonstration of antigen /antibody
- CFT
- SAT
- ELISA
- DIA
- Isolation of bacteria
- Demonstration of organisms in tissue sections using special stains.

Haemorrhagic Septicemia

Haemorrhagic septicemia is a highly contagious and infectious disease of animals caused by *Pasteurella multocida* and *Mannheimia hemolytica* and characterized by oedematous swelling in neck region,dyspnoea, pneumonia and wide spread haemorrhage in visceral organs (Fig.2.5).

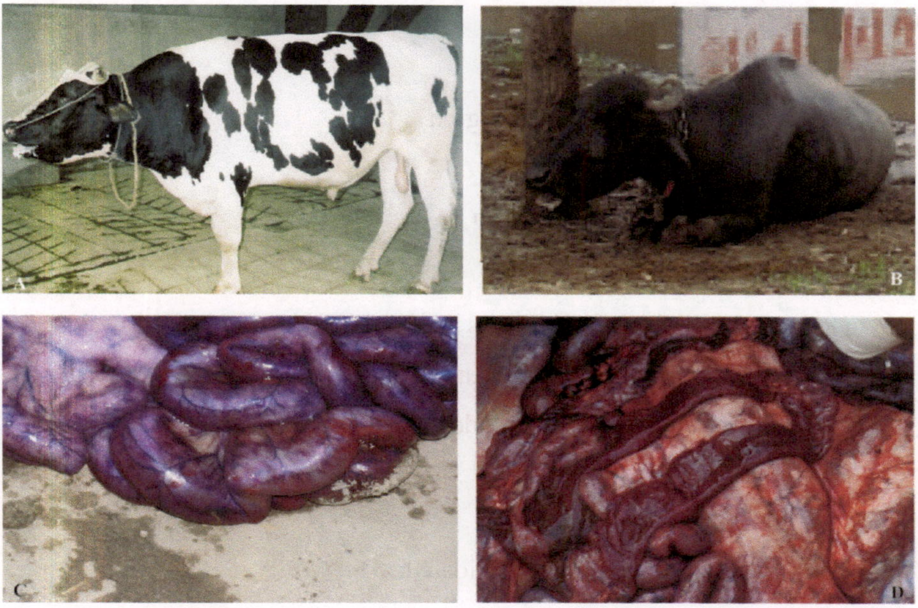

Fig. 2.5: Haemorrhagic Septaecemia in- A. Bull & B. Buffalo showing swelling in neck and briscket region alongwith dyspnoea, C. & D Intestinal haemorrhage.

Etiology

- *Pasteurella multocida*
- *Mannheimia hemolytica*

Pathogenesis

The disease spreads by ingestion of contaminated feed and water. The saliva of affected animals contains large number of organisms during the early stages of the disease. The organism is normal inhabitant in the terminal bronchioles and alveoli and it can't invade the lungs because of pulmonary defense but due to stress like malnutrition, long transportation, climatic changes, the organism become virulent and destroys the mononuclear leucocytes of bloods and macrophages of lungs. Due to death of macrophages vasoactive substances are released to cause inflammation and fibrin deposition. The other secondary invaders like PI-3 virus, bovine herpes virus and bacteria cause significant change. Death occurs due to hypoxia and toxaemia. It has been reported that primarily there is infection of PI-3 virus which is precipitated by bacteria resulting in septicemia.

Characteristic symptoms

- High fever(105-107°F)
- Oedema in throat and brisket region
- Dyspnoea
- Ghar –ghar sound on respiration

Macroscopic features

- Oedema consisting of gelatinous material in neck and brisket region
- Serosanguinous fluid in peritoneal and pleural cavity
- Swollen and enlarged lymph nodes
- Pericardial haemorrhage
- Haemorrhagic gastroenteritis
- Lungs are congested and consolidated "***Marbling***".

Microscopic features

- Fibrinous bronchopneumonia
- Congestion and haemorrhage in lymph nodes, spleen, liver, kidneys and myocardium
- Congestion and haemorrhage in intestinal mucosa and sub mucosa
- Infiltration of neutrophils, macrophages and lymphocytes.

Diagnosis

- Symptoms and lesions
- Demonstration of bipolar bacteria in blood smears on methylene blue staining
- Isolation of bacteria
- Immunodiagnostic tests for demonstration of antigen /antibody
- ELISA

Black Quarter

Black Quarter is an acute disease of cattle and sheep caused by *Clostrium chauvei* and characterized by lameness, hot painful swelling in thigh muscles producing crepitating sound on pressure and accumulation of serosanguinous fluid in affected area (Fig. 2.6).

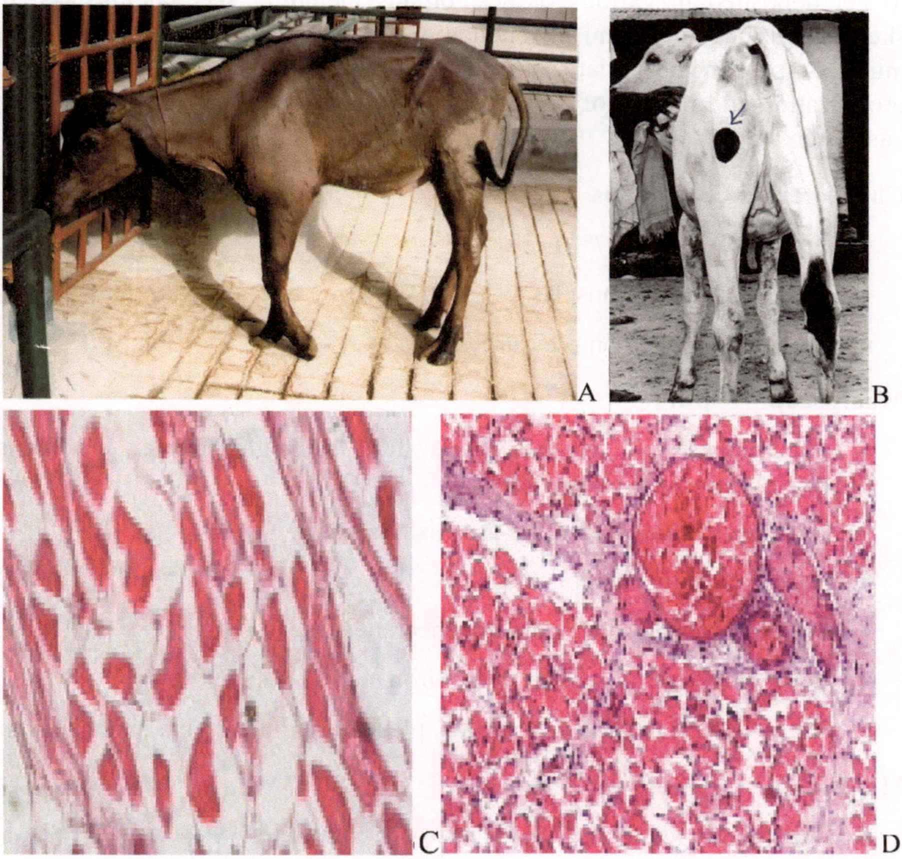

Fig. 2.6: Black quarter affecting: **A**. Shoulder, **B**. Thigh muscles and **C & D** Oedema, congestion and infiltration of leucocytes in affected muscles.

Etiology

- *Clostridium chauvei*
- Gram positive, anaerobe

Pathogenesis

The organism is transmitted through contaminated soil. Route of entry is through alimentary tract mucosa after ingestion of spores in contaminated feed. In case of sheep, the disease is generally occurs by wound infection.

After ingestion and germination of the spores, the bacteria multiplies in the intestines and crosses the intestinal mucosa and enters in general circulation to get deposited in various tissues/ organs including skeletal muscles. In skeletal muscles the organism remains in dormant stage until damage to the muscle sets up an appropriate anaerobic environment for their germination and proliferation and release of certain toxins locally which causes necrosis and gas gangrene of muscles.

Characteristic symptoms

- High fever (104-107°F)
- Swelling in thigh muscles
- Crepitating sound on pressure

Macroscopic features

- Accumulation of serosanguinous fluid in thigh muscles producing crepitating sound on pressure
- The affected area looks like greenish or bluish
- Oedema of subcutaneous tissue
- Affected muscles have porous appearance due to presence of gas
- Black colour of muscles is due to iron sulfide (FeS)
- Fibrino haemorrhagic pericarditis, pleurisy and ulcerative endocarditis.

Microscopic features

- Degeneration and coagulative necrosis of muscles
- Streaks of haemorrhage between fibers
- Presence of 'Rod' shaped bacteria, oedema and infiltration of leucocytes.

Diagnosis

- Symptoms and lesions
- Demonstration of Gram positive bacteria in exudate
- Isolation of bacteria
- Immunodiagnostic tests for demonstration of antigen /antibody
- ELISA
- Demonstration of organism in muscle tissue section using special stains.

Enterotoxaemia

Enterotoxaemia is an acute disease of sheep, goat and camel caused by *Clostridium perfringens* and characterized by endocardial haemorrhage, gastroenteritis and pulpy kidneys.

Etiology

- *Clostridium perfringens* type D-sheep
- *Clostridium perfringens* type A-camel.

Pathogenesis

The organism is normal inhabitant of gut in animals. When there is anaerobic condition develops in gut due to over feeding, this organism starts proliferation and production of toxins. The toxins are readily absorbed through stomach and intestines to cause disease in animals.

Characteristic symptoms

- Over filled stomach
- Sudden mortality
- Hyperglycemia

Macroscopic features

- Enlarged pulpy kidneys
- Congestion of abomasum and intestines
- Haemorrhage on endocardium and pericardium
- Congestion and oedema of lungs.

Microscopic features

- Cloudy swelling and necrosis of tubular epithelium in kidneys
- Congestion in liver, spleen and intestines
- Endocardial haemorrhage
- Oedema in lungs.

Diagnosis

- History of over feeding
- Symptoms and lesions

- Demonstration of toxin in intestinal/ stomach contents on mouse inoculation test
- Isolation and identification of causative organism.

Braxy

Braxy is an acute fatal disease of sheep caused by *Clostridium septicum* and characterized by oedema, necrosis and haemorrhage in abomasum (Fig.2.7).

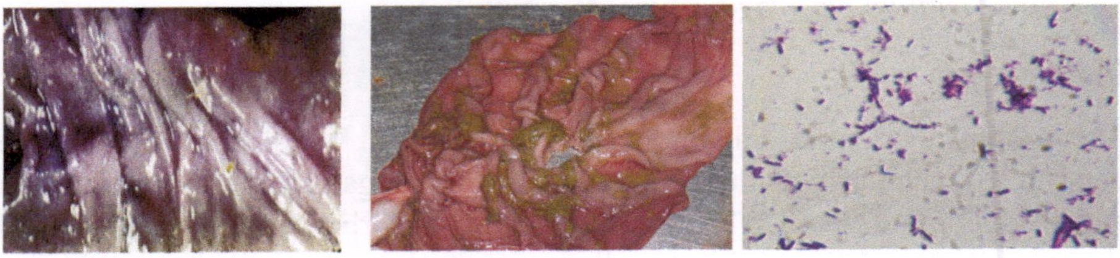

A B C

Fig. 2.7: Braxy in sheep- A.& B.Oedema and congestion in abomasum and C. Clostridium sp in impression smear from abomasum.

Etiology

- *Clostridium septicum*

Pathogenesis

It is a soil borne infection and mostly occurs in sheep vaccinated with enterotoxaemia vaccine. The organism gets entry through ingestion of spores. The ingested spores are localized in stomach and germinate under anaerobic conditions due to over feeding of lush green feed or high amount of grains leading to abomasitis.

Characteristic symptoms

- Over filled stomach
- Sudden mortality
- History of enterotoxaemia vaccination

Macroscopic features

- Oedema of abomasal folds
- Congestion and haemorrhage in abomasum
- Necrosis of abomasal mucosa
- Congestion and necrosis in intestines.

Microscopic features

- Congestion and haemorrhage of abomasal mucosa
- Presence of 'Rod' shaped organism in mucosal epithelium of abomasum
- Necrosis and presence of ulcers in abomasal mucosa.

Diagnosis

- History of over feeding and enterotoxaemia vaccination
- Symptoms and lesions
- Demonstration of toxin in intestinal/ stomach contents on mouse inoculation test
- Isolation and identification of bacteria

Tetanus

Tetanus is a bacterial disease of animals caused by the toxins of clostridia and characterized by prolonged spasmodic contractions of muscles, stiffness and immobilization. It is also known as ***"lock jaw"*** (Fig.2.8).

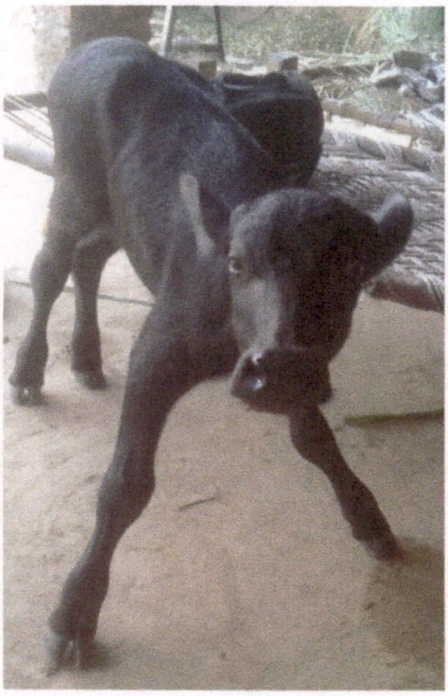

Fig. 2.8: Tetanus in a calf showing stiffness of the muscles

Etiology

- *Clostridium tetani*
- Gram positive, anaerobe, rod shaped, produces toxins

Pathogenesis

It occurs as a sequel to a wound that allows the growth of anaerobic *Clostridium tetani*, which releases neurotoxins. This neurotoxin fixes the gray matter of the brain and spinal cord and causes stiffness of muscles leading to asphyxia and death.

Clinical Symptoms

- Convulsions
- Immobilization
- Stiffness of muscles
- Lock jaw

Macroscopic features

- Presence of wound or history of wound.
- Stiffness of muscles

Microscopic features

- Gram positive organism in wound.
- Necrosis in muscles and gray matter of brain.

Diagnosis

- Symptoms and lesions
- Presence of wound and bacteria

Swine Erysepalas

It is an important disease of pigs caused by a Gram-positive bacteria and characterized by arthritis, vegetative endocarditis and rhomboid shaped erythematous skin lesions. It is also known as ***"diamond skin disease"*** (Fig.2.9).

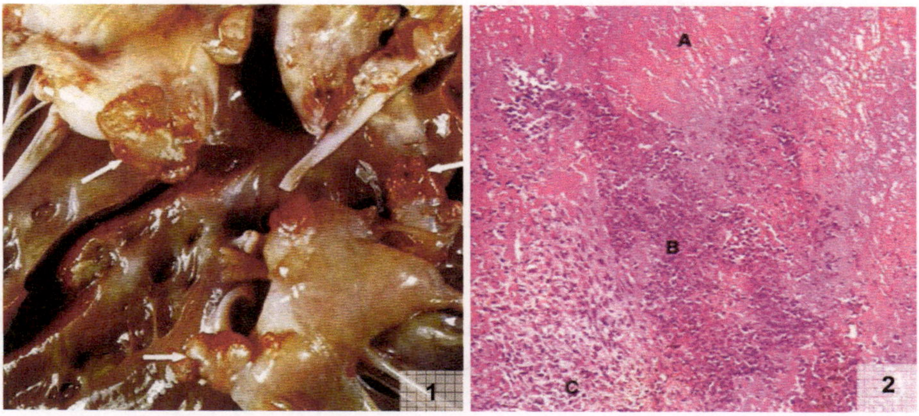

Fig. 2.9: Swine erysepalas- (1) Vegetable endocarditis, (2) Microscopic features of vegetative endocarditis A. Layer of platelets and fibrin, B. Layer of leukocytes (neutrophils) and C. Chronic inflammatory cells in myofibrils.

Etiology

- *Erysepalothrix rhusiopathie*
- Gram-positive, rod shaped, pleomorphic

Pathogenesis

Infection enters through skin or ingestion and causes bacteremia or septicemia. The organism then localizes in joints, skin and heart valves to produce lesions.

Clinical Symptoms

- Arthritis
- Erythema on skin, later sloughing of skin and patches on abdomen.

Macroscopic features

- Arthritis
- Erythema or sloughing of skin
- Vegetative endocarditis- nodular mass of over growth on valves
- Hypertrophy of left ventricle

Microscopic features

- Infiltration of lymphocytes in joint capsules
- Fibrinous exudate with necrosis, leucocytic infilteration and colonies of bacteria in heart lesions.

- Necrosis in skin sections.

Diagnosis

- Symptoms and lesions
- Isolation of bacteria
- Demonstration of bacteria in tissue sections using special stains.

Listeriosis

Listeriosis is an acute infectious disease of animals caused by *Listeria* sp. and characterized by congestion of meninges and brain, presence of micro abscess in brain and lymphocytic leptomeningitis.

Etiology

- *Listeria monocytogenes (L. ivanovi)*

Pathogenesis

Listeria is transmitted by ingestion of contaminated materials. Silage is considered as one of the important organism. Besides, it is normal inhabitant of bowl of many animals. There are certain predisposing factors including nutritional deficiencies, silage feeding, weather change and long duration flood etc. The organism penetrates the epithelial cells of intestines, conjunctiva, urinary bladder etc. The organism has a lucein rich protein on their surface known as internalins, which is required for penetration into epithelial cells. Internalins bind with E-cadherin on host epithelial cells. They multiply in epithelial cells, destroy the cells and are released then they are phagocytosed by macrophages and multiply there. The activated macrophages can phagocyte and kill bacteria. The centripetal movement of bacteria in trigeminal nerve eventually make them to reach medulla oblongata. The listeria organism is excreted in faeces in animals even in absence of disease.

Characteristic symptoms

- High fever(105-107°F)
- Circling movements
- Abortion
- Torticollis

Macroscopic features

- Congestion and/or haemorrhage in meninges
- Foci of softening / micro abscess in medulla
- Small necrotic foci / abscess in visceral organs.

Microscopic features

- Microabscess in brain
- Infiltration of mononuclear cells and neutrophils
- Perivascular cuffing by lymphocytes, eosinophils, histiocytes and neutrophils
- Softening of brain / liquifactive necrosis.

Diagnosis

- Symptoms and lesions
- Isolation and identification of bacteria
- Immunodiagnostic tests for demonstration of antigen /antibody
- ELISA
- Demonstration of bacteria in tissue sections using special stains.

Salmonellosis

Salmonellosis is an infectious disease of calves, lambs and piglets caused by *Salmonella* sp. and characterized by septicemia, wide spread haemorrhage on visceral organs, typhoid nodules in liver and haemorrhagic enteritis.

Etiology

- *Salmonella enteritidis* var. Typhimurium (*S.* Typhimurium)
- *Salmonella enteritidis* var. Dublin (*S.* Dublin)
- *Salmonella enteritidis* var. Cholaraesuis (*S.* Cholaraesuis)

Pathogenesis

It is transmitted horizontally by direct or indirect contact. Infection is acquired by ingestion of materials contaminated with faeces of clinically ill animals. After entry, bacteria adhere to intestinal cells through fimbriae/pilli and colonize in small intestine then they penetrate enterocytes (intestinal cells) for further multiplication. They cross lamina propria and continue to proliferate both free and within macrophages and are transported to mesenteric lymph nodes. Further multiplication leads to septicaemia and spread of the bacteria to various organs/ tissues like spleen, liver, meninges, brain and joints. It may cause mild enteritis to fatal enteritis with septicemia.

Characteristic symptoms

- Fever(102-105°F)
- Weakness, icterus, anemia
- Diarrhoea, melena
- Dehydration

Macroscopic features

- Haemorrhage in intestines
- Petechiae on kidneys "***Turkey egg appearance***"
- Oedema of spleen and lymph nodes
- Button ulcers in intestines of piglets
- Focal necrosis and reactive granuloma in liver "***Typhoid nodules***".

Microscopic features

- Necrosis and desquamation of intestinal mucosal epithelium
- Necrosis in liver and infiltration by neutrophils, macrophages and lymphocytes
- Congestion and oedema in spleen and lymph nodes.

Diagnosis

- Symptoms and lesions
- Isolation of bacteria
- Immunodiagnostic tests for demonstration of antigen /antibody
- SAT
- ELISA
- Demonstration of bacteria in tissue sections using special stains.

Colibacillosis

Colibacillosis is an infectious disease of new born animals caused by *E. coli* and characterized by enteritis, swelling of lymph nodes and peyer's patches, pneumonia and haemorrhage on endocardium.

Etiology

- *Escherichia coli*

Pathogenesis

The disease is transmitted through contaminated feed and water. Discharges of aborted foetus, vaginal discharges, umbilical infection and intrauterine infection may act as source of infection for newly born animals. The colonization of organism in gut depends on the immune status animals. The cell wall of *E.coli* consists of lipopolysaccharide which causes fever mediated through the production of host cytokines including TNF and IL-1. *E.coli* also secretes substances that suppresses phagocytosis by neutrophils. The endotoxins secreted by *E.coli* is an ADP- ribosyltransferase which generate excess c- AMP to cause diarrhoea and dehydration.

Characteristic symptoms

- Fever(103-106°F)
- Diarrhoea, dehydration
- Nasal discharges
- Naval ill

Macroscopic features

- Swollen umblicus
- Swelling of joints
- Suppurative nephritis
- Congestion and haemorrhage in intestines
- Congestion of lungs and mesenteric lymph nodes
- Haemorrhage in endocardium.

Microscopic features

- Necrosis and desquamation of mucosal epithelium in intestine
- Infiltration of neutrophils and mononuclear cells

- Infiltration of neutrophils in kidneys forming micro abscess
- Catarrhal bronchopneumonia
- Congestion and reactive hyperplasia in lymph nodes.

Diagnosis

- Symptoms and lesions
- Isolation of bacteria
- Immunodiagnostic tests for demonstration of antigen /antibody
- ELISA
- Demonstration of organisms in tissue sections using special stains.

Strangles

Strangles is an acute infectious disease of horses caused by streptococci and characterized by abscess in pharyngeal and maxillary lymph nodes, pericarditis, pleurisy, suppurative pneumonia, presence of abscess on liver, kidneys and spleen (Fig.2.10).

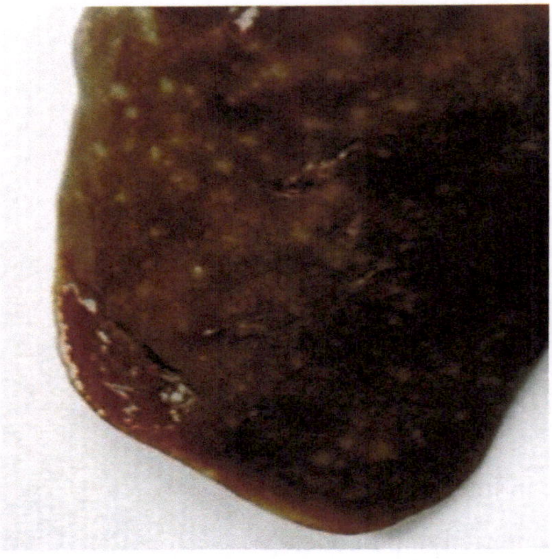

Fig. 2.10: Strangles in horse- Miliary abscess in liver.

Etiology

- *Streptococcus equi*

Pathogenesis

The disease spreads through inhalation; the most important source of infection is nasal discharge. The bacteria reaches on pharyngeal and nasal mucosa and causes acute pharyngitis and rhinitis. Drainage to lymph nodes leads to formation of abscess. Guttural pouches are filled with pus. Then infection spreads in other organs and causes suppuration in kidneys, brain, liver, spleen, tendon sheath and joints. After an attack, strangles has subsided and purpura haemorrhagica may develop due to the development of sensitivity to streptococcal proteins.

Characteristic symptoms

- Fever(104-107°F)
- Abscess in throat region
- Dyspnoea

Macroscopic features

- Abscess in pharyngeal and sub maxillary lymph nodes
- Abscess in liver, kidneys and spleen
- Suppurative pericarditis
- Suppurative pneumonia
- Empyema.

Microscopic features

- Infiltration of neutrophils in liver, kidneys, spleen, pericardium and lungs
- Degeneration and necrosis in liver along with accumulation of neutrophils
- Lymphoid depletion in spleen.

Diagnosis

- Symptoms and lesions
- Isolation of bacteria
- Immunodiagnostic tests for demonstration of antigen /antibody
- ELISA
- Demonstration of organisms in tissue sections using special stains.

Glanders

Glanders is an infectious disease of equines caused by *Pseudomonas* sp. characterized by ulcers in nasal passage, miliary nodules in lungs, oedema of lymph nodes, lymphangitis and lymphadenitis (Fig.2.11).

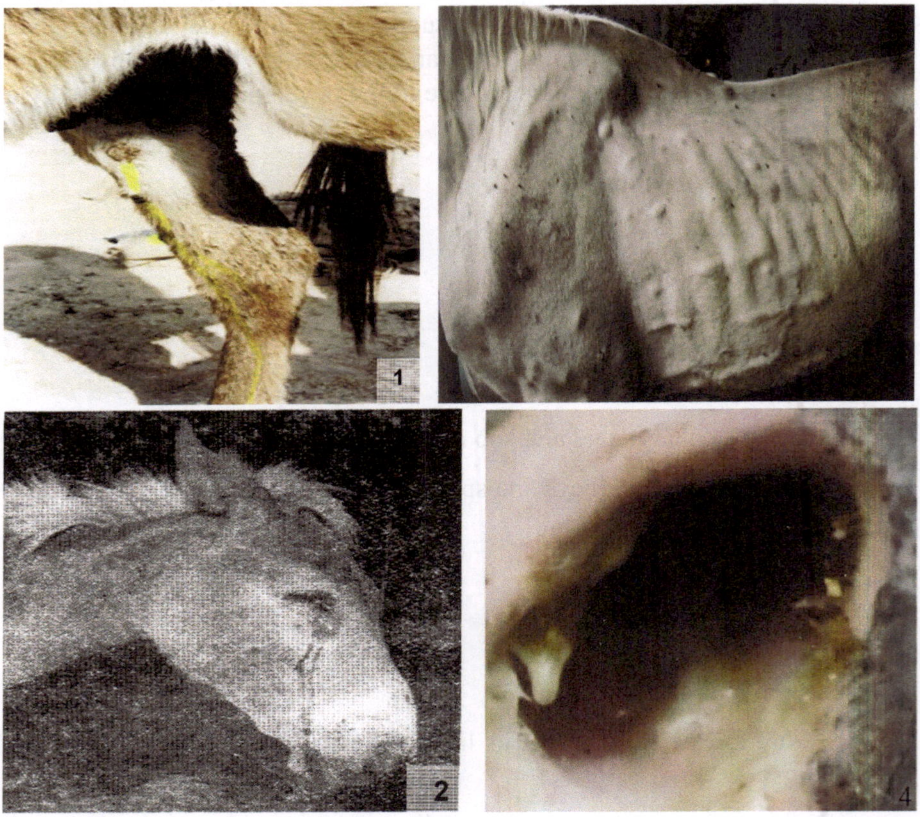

Fig. 2.11: Glanders in horse- (1) Farcy lesions in medial portion of hind leg, (2) Mallein- IDP test showing conjunctivitis and ocular discharges, 3.Lymphadenitis and 4. Ulcer in external nares and purulent nasal discharge.

Etiology

- *Pseudomonas mallei*

Pathogenesis

The disease is transmitted through ingestion of contaminated feed and water and also through utensils particularly watering troughs, contaminated by nasal discharge/ sputum. Rarely spread through direct contact or grooming tools.

Spread through inhalation can also occur. The organism invades the intestinal wall and causes septicaemia (acute form) or bacteraemia (chronic form). The organism may invade the regional lymph nodes by pharyngeal lymph nodes and proliferate there. The respiratory mucosa and lungs are most commonly affected but disseminated lesions may occur. Nasal involvement is indicated by a copious and persistent nasal discharge. In cutaneous form there is development of lesions along the lymphatics resulting in lymphangitis and lymphadenitis.

Characteristic symptoms

- Fever(103-105°F)
- Dyspnoea
- Discharge of pus from lymph vessels and lymph nodes
- Ulcer in nasal passage

Macroscopic features

- Abscess in superficial lymph nodes and discharge of oily pus from lymph vessels in hind legs
- Abscess in lungs and liver
- Pleurisy with purulent exudate
- Ulcers and deposition of purulent exudate in nasal passage
- Enlargement of lymph nodes
- Punched out ulcers in lungs.

Microscopic features

- Centrally aggregates of neutrophils surrounded by histiocytes in lungs
- Infiltration of neutrophils in and around necrotic foci in liver, kidneys and intestines.
- Oedema in lymph nodes

Diagnosis

- Symptoms and lesions
- Mallein testing of equines
- Isolation of bacteria

- Immunodiagnostic tests for demonstration of antigen /antibody
- ELISA
- CFT
- Demonstration of organism in tissue sections using special stains.

Anthrax

Anthrax is an acute septicemic disease of animals caused by *Bacillus* sp. and characterized by sudden death, absence of rigor mortis, tary colour blood from natural openings and widespread haemorrhage (Fig.2.12).

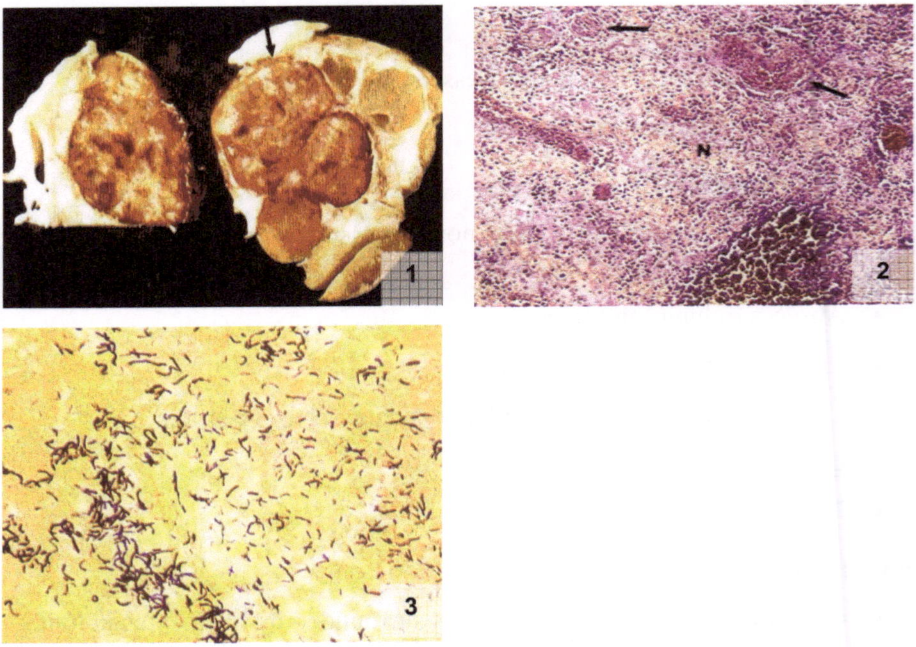

Fig. 2.12: Anthrax in animals-(1) Haemorrhagic and necrotic lesions in lymph nodes, (2) Microscopic features including necrosis in lymph node and (3) Anthrax bacilli in lymph node

Etiology

- *Bacillus anthracis*

Pathogenesis

The infection occurs through ingestion or inhalation of spores/ vegetative forms of the organism or entry of bacteria through broken skin. After entry the spores germinate and localize for multiplication and spread by means of lymphatics to lymph nodes and then in blood stream, causing severe septicaemia. The bacteria possesses both capsule and exotoxin. Due to presence of capsule phagocytic cells become unable to destroy them. The exotoxin is lethal in nature, it causes oedema and tissue damage. The exotoxin has 3 components-

1. Oedema factor (EF) or factor I is adenyl cyclase which causes increase in cellular c-AMP level that causes electrolyte and fluid loss.
2. Protective antigen (PA) or factor II is a fragment of exotoxin and has anti-phagocytic activity.
3. Lethal factor (LF) or factor III stimulates macrophages for production of oxidizing radicals and cytokines. Mainly IL-1 and TNF- α, which induce shock and death.

Characteristic symptoms

- High fever(105-107°F)
- Haemorrhage from natural orifices
- Dyspnoea
- Tary colour blood
- Sudden mortality up to 90%

Macroscopic features

- Post mortem examination of animals suspected for anthrax should not be conducted.
- Blood smear examined for anthrax bacilli
- Discharge of blood from vagina, anus and mouth
- Tary colour of blood
- Enlargement of spleen
- Widespread haemorrhage on serous surfaces of visceral organs
- Subcutaneous oedema

Microscopic features

- Anthrax bacilli and spores in blood smear
- Spleen shows haemorrhage and accumulation of blood in red pulp
- Haemorrhage in lymph nodes, liver, lungs and kidneys

- Degenerative and necrotic changes in kidneys and liver.

Diagnosis

- Symptoms and lesions
- Demonstration of bacteria in blood smear
- Immunodiagnostic tests for demonstration of antigen /antibody
- ELISA
- AGPT (Ascoli test)
- Animal inoculation test causes death of mouse within 24 hrs.

Campylobacteriosis

Campylobacteriosis is an infectious disease of cattle and sheep caused by *Campylobacter* sp. and characterized by early abortion, suppurative metritis, cervicitis and vaginitis.

Etiology

- *Campylobacter foetus*

Pathogenesis

The bacteria is natural inhabitant of reproductive tract of bovines. In case of males, it is confined to prepucial cavity and mucosa of glans penis and distal portion of urethra. In females, lumen of vagina, cervix, uterus and oviduct harbor the bacteria. Infection spreads through coitus or AI due to use of infected semen. From bull to bull transmission occurs through artificial vagina at breeding centers. After entry in females, the bacteria multiplies in the cervix and reaches to uterine horn and oviduct within 7-14 days. In the cervix, the organism metabolizes amino acids and other organic acids. The organism is protected from phagocytes because it is covered with mucous. This organism causes abortion at 5 month of gestation because the organism impairs the supply of oxygen and some nutrients (amino acids) required for implantation of embryo leading to abortion.

Characteristic symptoms

- Abortion in mid gestation (5 month)
- Mucopurulent vaginal discharge
- Retention of placenta

Macroscopic features

- Abortions at 4-5 month of gestation
- Purulent exudate in uterine discharges- yellowish
- Congestion of vagina
- Oedema in foetus
- Necrotic foci in liver
- Oedematous placenta.

Microscopic features

- Infiltration of neutrophils, macrophages and lymphocytes in uterine mucosa
- Enlargement of uterine glands
- Necrosis in placenta
- Suppurative endometritis, cervicitis and vaginitis.

Diagnosis

- Symptoms and lesions
- Isolation of bacteria
- Immunodiagnostic tests for demonstration of antigen /antibody
- ELISA
- Demonstration of organisms in tissue sections using special stains.

Actinobacillosis

Actinobacillosis is a disease of cattle caused by *Actinobacillus* sp. and characterized by granulomatous lesions in tongue, lymph nodes and presence of colony of organism (palisade of Indian club like structures) in between the inflammatory exudate. This is also known as ***wooden tongue*** (Fig.2.13).

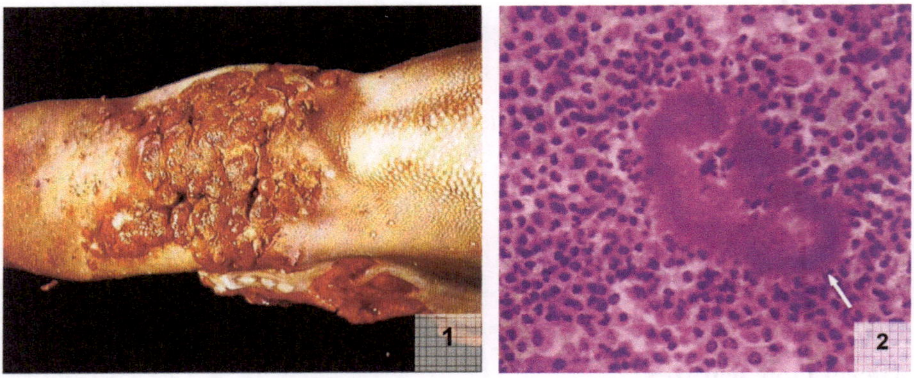

Fig. 2.13: Actinobacillosis-(1) Hardening of tongue, (2) Presence of sulfur granules (arrow) in granulomatous lesion.

Etiology

- *Actinobacillus legniresei*

Pathogenesis

The organism is normally present in the oral cavity of cattle and sheep. Infection occurs when there is traumatic injury of oral mucosa. When condition become favourable to the causative organism due to injury, it reaches to regional lymph nodes and nasal mucosa. The organism has affinity with soft tissues and thus affects soft tissue of head and neck. There is acute inflammatory changes and subsequent granulomatous reaction including necrosis and suppuration.

Characteristic symptoms

- Anorexia, pain in tongue due to hardening
- Sporadic occurrence
- Drooling of saliva

Macroscopic features

- Enlargement of tongue due to granuloma formation.
- Nodular lesions may also appear in rumen, skin, lungs and liver
- Flooding of pus from lesions present in tongue.

Microscopic features

- Presence of colony of organism palisade of Indian club like structures surrounded by neutrophils, mononuclear cells and lymphocytes

- Such lesions are surrounded by fibrous tissue
- Muscle tissue of tongue is replaced by fibrous tissue.

Diagnosis

- Symptoms and lesions
- Isolation of bacteria
- Demonstration of organisms/colony in tissue sections.

Actinomycosis

Actinomycosis is a disease of cattle, buffaloes and camels caused by *Actinomyces* sp. and characterized by suppurative osteomyelitis of mandible and Miliary nodules in lungs. This is also known as ***lumpy jaw*** (Fig.2.14).

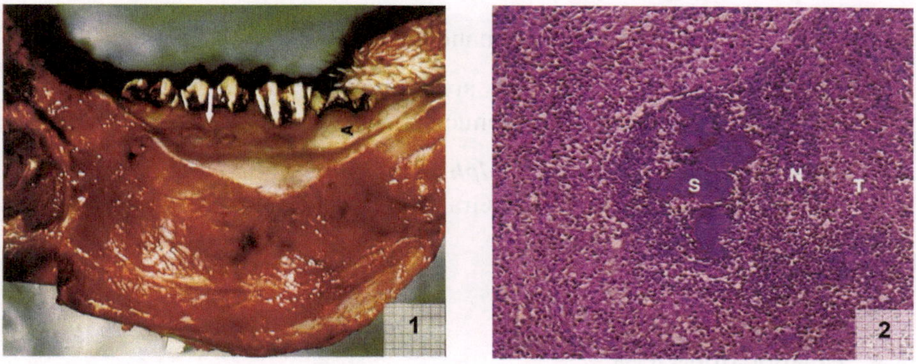

Fig. 2.14: Actinomycosis- (1) Abscess and chronic granulomatous lesions (A) and (2) Sulfur granules surrounded by neutrophils and other inflammatory cells.

Etiology

- *Actinomyces bovis*

Pathogenesis

The causative organism is a normal inhabitant of the bovine buccal cavity and infection occurs through wounds in buccal mucosa due to sharp edged objects. After entry from buccal cavity, it causes rarefaction of bone followed by osteomyelitis characterized by chronic suppurative and granulomatous reaction.

Characteristic symptoms

- Anorexia due to pain in jaw
- Abscess in mandible and swelling of jaw
- Discharging of pus from lesion

Macroscopic features

- Lumpy jaw
- Swelling of jaw at mandible
- Miliary nodules in lungs and mammary gland
- Discharging of pus from jaw.

Microscopic features

- Suppurative osteomyelitis of mandible
- Central liquifactive necrosed area which is having colonies of the organism surrounded by mononuclear and lymphocytic cells
- Colonies are known as ***sulphur granules***, bigger in size than actinobacillosis and may take Gram positive stain.

Diagnosis

- Symptoms and lesions
- Isolation of bacteria
- Demonstration of organisms/colony in tissue sections using special stains.

Botriomycosis (Staphylococcosis)

Botriomycosis is an infectious disease of animals caused by staphylococci and characterized by suppurative granulomatous lesions in udder, jaw, shoulder or sternal region (Fig.2.15).

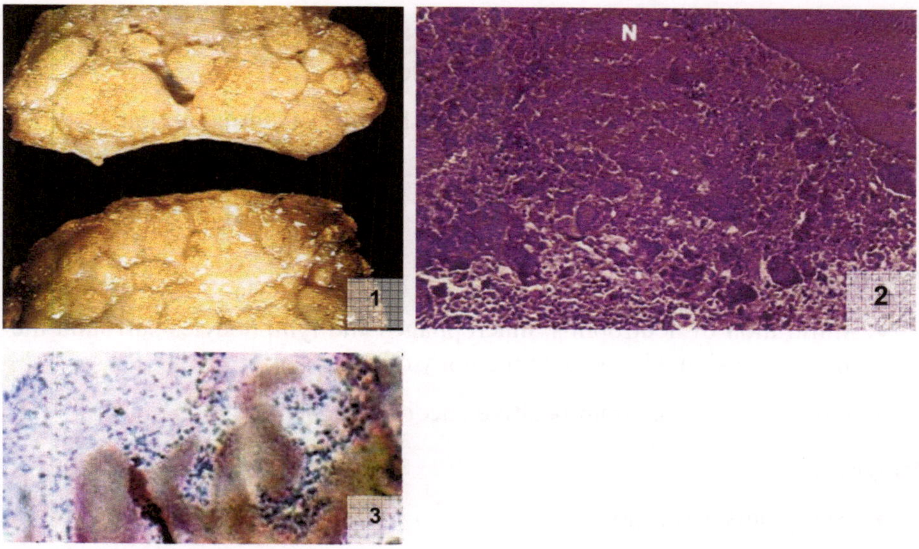

Fig. 2.15: Staphylococcosis- in mammary gland- (1) Lobules of gland surrounded by chronic inflammatory tissue, (2) Caseative necrosis (N) surrounded by chronic inflammatory reaction (T) and (3) Presence of staphylococcosis colonies in between inflammatory cells.

Etiology

- *Staphylococcus aureus*

Pathogenesis

The causative agent is transmitted through contamination of infected animals. The organism possesses number of virulent factors which include surface proteins for adherence, enzyme for protein degradation and toxins for host cell damage. *S. aureus* has receptors for fibrinogen, fibrinolectin and vintronectin on their surface through which it binds with host endothelial cells. The toxin produced by bacteria contains coagulase, fibrinolysins, hyaluronidase, hemolysins and endotoxins. The lipases destroy the skin surface and thus help the bacteria in abscessation.

Characteristic symptoms

- Hardening of udder
- Papillary projections from jaw
- Yellow pus discharge from lesion

Macroscopic features

- Hard and nodular enlargement of udder
- Hard over growth in lower jaw or at shoulder or sternal region
- Yellow pus discharges from lesions
- Enlargement of lymph nodes.

Microscopic features

- Infiltration of neutrophils, macrophages and lymphocytes surround the necrotic lesion which contain colony of organism
- On Gram's stain, Gram positive cocci are seen.

Diagnosis

- Symptoms and lesions
- Isolation of bacteria
- Demonstration of organisms in tissue sections using special stains.

Necrobacillosis

Necrobacillosis is an infectious disease of animals caused by *Spherophorus necrophorus* and characterized by necrosis of liver, foot rot, diphtheria and enteritis (Fig.2.16).

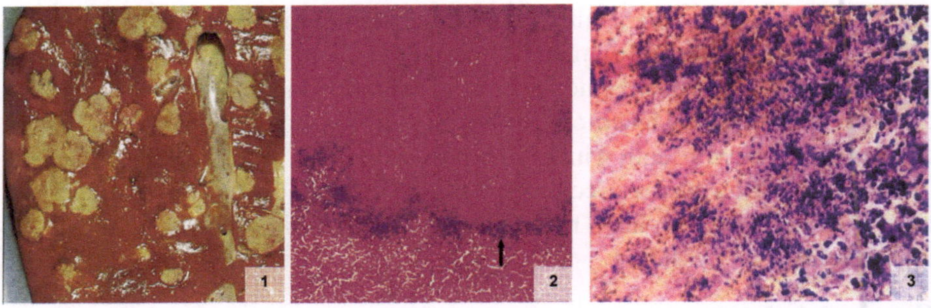

Fig. 2.16: Necrobacillosis- (1) Coagulative necrosis in liver, (2) Zone of inflammation dividing areas of necrosis and from normal liver parenchyma and (3) Dark coloured organisms in tissue.

Etiology

- *Spherophorus necrophorus*

Pathogenesis

The causative organism is a common inhabitant of the oral cavity. It produces a variety of toxins including exo- and endtoxins which are the cause of necrosis, oedema, laryngitis and dyspnoea. There is formation of diphtheritic membrane over oral mucosa. In sheep it causes abscess formation in foot.

Characteristic symptoms

- Nasal discharge
- Coughing
- Sneezing
- Diarrhoea
- Lameness

Macroscopic features

- Presence of diphtheritic membrane of tongue and pharynx in calves
- On removal of diphtheritic membrane, ulcer is left
- Necrotic areas in trachea
- Suppurative pneumonia
- Necrotic lesions in esophagus, rumen, abomasum, liver, spleen and heart
- Necrotic lesions and gangrenous foot.

Microscopic features

- Necrosis and infiltration of neutrophils in liver
- Necrosis and bronchopneumonia in lungs
- Necrosis of epithelium, ulcer and infiltration of neutrophils in tongue
- Congestion in lungs and liver.

Diagnosis

- Symptoms and lesions
- Isolation of bacteria
- Immunodiagnostic tests for demonstration of antigen /antibody
- ELISA

- Demonstration of organisms in tissue sections using special stains.

Nocardiosis

Nocardiosis is a bacterial disease of animals caused by gram-positive bacteria and characterized by pneumonia, mastitis, lymphangitis and lymphadenitis. This is also known as "***Bovine Farcy***" (Fig.2.17).

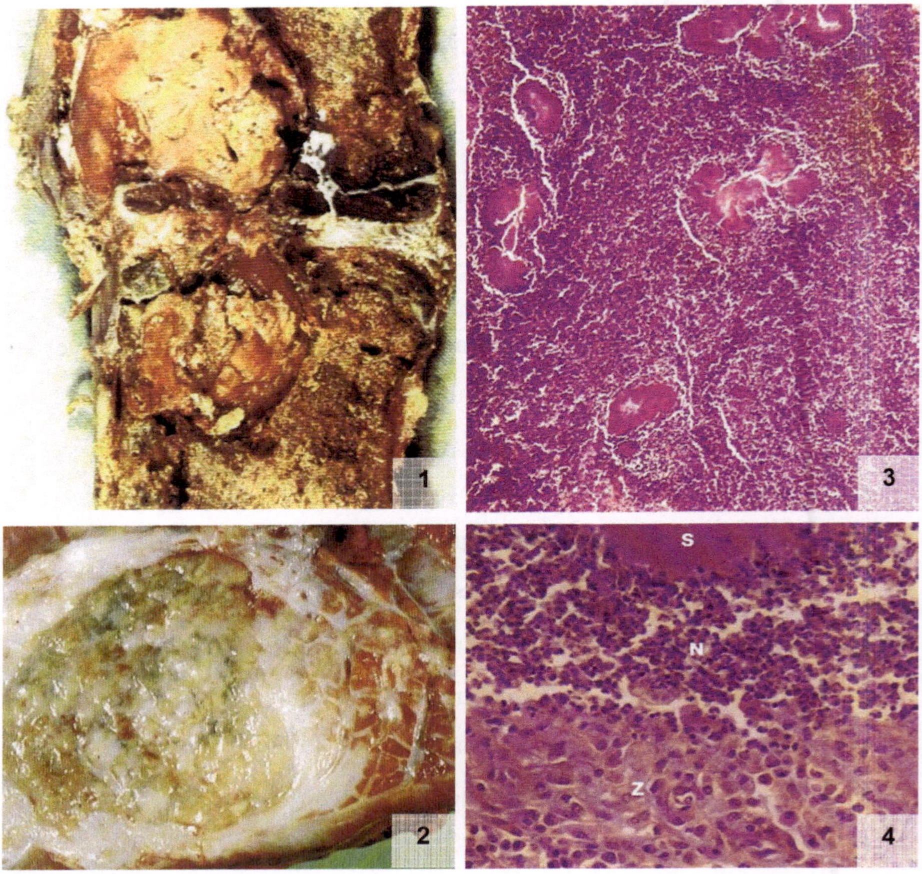

Fig. 2.17: Nocardiosis- (1) Abscess in vertebrae, (2) Narcardial abscess in lung, (3) Presence of sulfur granules in between inflammatory cells and (4) Sulfur granules (S), Zone of neutrophils (N) and Zone of proliferative tissue (Z).

Etiology

- *Nocardia asteroids*
- Gram-positive, acid fast, aerobic, filamentus

Pathogenesis

Organism enter via soil contamination of wounds and causes local subcutaneous oedema which also spreads to lymph nodes. Lesions may break skin to form abscess and sinuses connecting two abscesses. This is pyogranuloma formation.

Clinical Symptoms

- Purulent nasal discharge
- Discharge from lymphatics and lymph nodes "***Farcy***"
- Mastitis and abortion

Macroscopic features

- Granulomatous lesions in lungs
- Mastitis- hardness of udder
- Lymphatics discharging pus
- Enlargement of lymph nodes, spleen and liver with abscess.

Microscopic features

- Granulomatous lesion in lungs- in central area acid-fast organism surrounded by neutrophils, macrophages, lymphocytes and giant cells.
- Tangled colonies of organism in necrotic debris.
- Purulent exudate

Diagnosis

- Symptoms and lesions
- Isolation and identification of bacteria
- Demonstration of organisms in tissue sections using special stains.

Pseudotuberculosis

Pseudotuberculosis is a chronic disease of sheep, goat and camel caused by *Corynebacterium pseudotuberculosis* and characterized by pyogranulomatous lesions in lymph nodes. This is also known as caseous lymphadenitis (Fig.2.18).

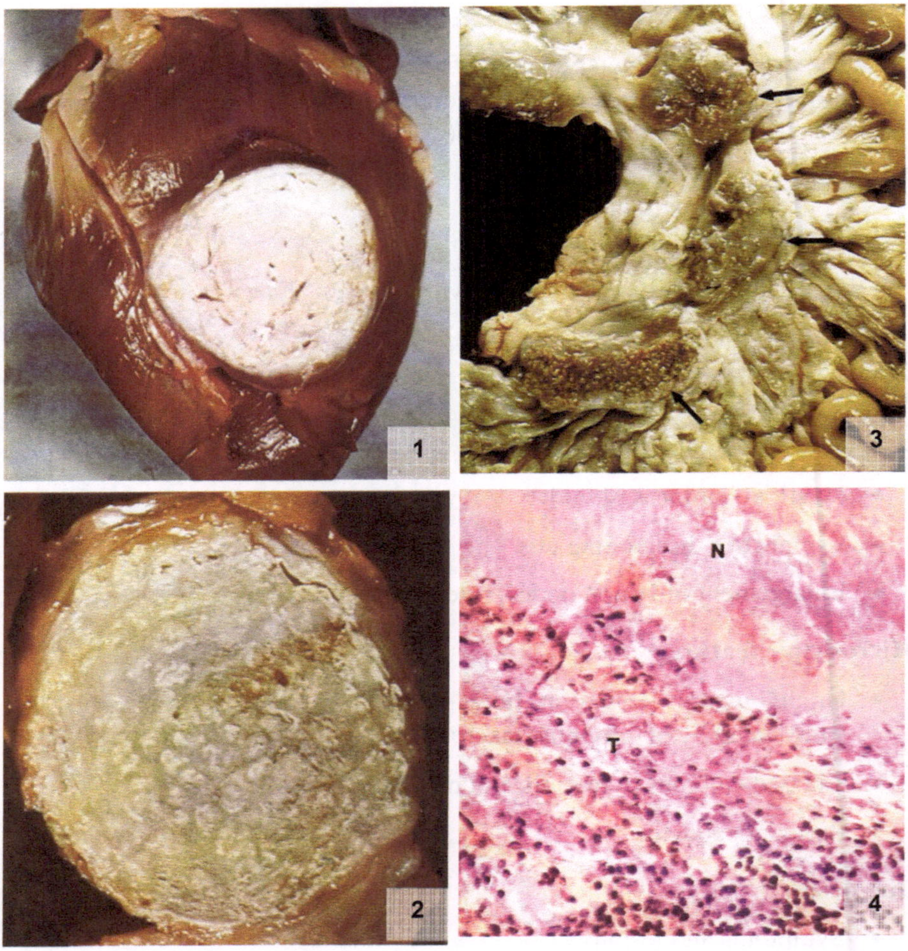

Fig. 2.18: Caseous lymphadenitis in sheep- (1) Caseation in heart, (2) Caseation necrosis in lymph node, (3) Caseative necrosis in mesenteric lymphnode and (4) Caseation (N) surrounded by chronic inflammatory cells.

Etiology

- *Corynebacterium pseudotuberculosis* or *C. ovis*
- Gram-positive, diphtheroid bacillus

Pathogenesis

Infection enters through abraded skin or oral mucous membrane and involves the local lymph nodes. The organism is intracellular and survive within macrophages due to presence of a toxic lipid. It terms absecess and caseation in lymph nodes, lungs, liver, kidney, brain, skin and spinal cord.

Clinical Symptoms

- Enlargement of lymph nodes
- Discharge of thick green pus from lymph nodes
- Nodular lesions on skin (camels)
- Paraplegia/paralysis of hind legs

Macroscopic features

- Enlargement of lymph nodes
- Nodules on skin
- Caseous mass on cut of lesion, onion like concentric laminated mass
- Discharge of pus

Microscopic features

- Caseous necrosis surrounded by epithelioid cells, lymphocytes and covered by fibrous connective tissue
- Concentrically laminated mass with no giant cells
- Calcification

Diagnosis

- Symptoms and lesions
- Isolation and identification of causative organisms
- Demonstration of bacteria in tissue sections using special stains.

Yersiniosis

Yersiniosis is an infectious disease of animals caused by *Yersimia* sp. and characterized by abortion in cattle, necrotic hepatitis and arteritis. This is often confused with brucella induced abortions in cattle as yersimia serologically cross reacts with brucella.

Etiology

- *Yersinia enterocolitica*
- *Yersinia pseudotuberculosis*

Pathogenesis

Yersinia have a protein 'invasin' on their cell wall which binds with host cell integrins that helps in attachment and multiplication of organism inside the host cells. It causes necrosis, pus formation and formation of nodules in liver. This organism also causes placentitis leading to abortion.

Clinical Symptoms

- Abortion in cattle, sheep and goat
- Diarrhoea in pigs

Macroscopic features

- White/gray nodules on placenta and liver of aborted foetus
- Enteritis, ulcers in ileum
- Enlargement of mesenteric lymph nodes
- Necrotic foci in liver, spleen, lymph nodes and lungs

Microscopic features

- Necrotic lesions in liver surrounded by macrophages, lymphocytes, epithelioid cells and covered by fibrous capsule
- Necrosis in intestines, spleen, lymph nodes

Diagnosis

- Symptoms and lesions
- Isolation and identification of bacteria
- Immunodiagnostic tests for detection of antigen / antibody using SAT/ ELISA
- Demonstration of organisms in tissue sections using special stains.

Black Disease

Black disease is an infectious disease of sheep, cattle and buffaloes caused by *Clostridium nouyi* and characterized by necrotic hepatitis, hydropericardium and black discolouration of skin.

Etiology

- Clostridium nouyi
- Gram positive, rod, anaevobes
- Predisposed by *Fasciola hepatica* and *Fasciola gigantica* infection

Pathogenesis

The damage caused by metacerearial liver fluke in liver provides anaerobic environment favourable for growth of clostridial organism. The causative agent is normally present in intestine and it reaches in liver through metacercariae. The organism produces alpha and beta toxin which causes hepatic necrosis.

Clinical Symptoms

- Fever (105-107°F)
- Sudden death

Macroscopic features

- Focal or diffused streaks of necrosis in liver along the track of liver fluke migration
- Petechial on endocardium, epicardium with hydropericardium
- Black discolouration of subcutaneous / skin

Microscopic features

- Necrosis in liver, infiltration of neutrophils
- Congestion, haemorrhage
- Presence of gram positive rods in necrotic lesions

Diagnosis

- Symptoms and lesions
- Isolation and identification of organism and its toxin
- Demonstration of organisms in tissue sections/smear using special stains.

Botulism

Botulism is a fatal disease of animals caused by toxins of *Clostridium botulinum* and characterized by paralysis and sudden death.

Etiology

- *Clostridium botulinum*
- Neurotoxin C_1 and C_2
- Predisposing factor- phosphorus deficiency leading to pica.

Pathogenesis

Disease occurs on ingestion of contaminated materials such as bone chewing, bone meal, food of animal origin. The preformed toxins of botulinum in these materials act on peripheral nerve endings to cause their blockage leading to paralysis.

Clinical Symptoms

- Paralysis
- Sudden death

Macroscopic features

- No characteristics gross lesion

Microscopic features

- No characteristic gross lesion

Diagnosis

- History
- Symptoms
- Very difficult to establish diagnosis.

Oedema disease in pigs

Oedema disease in piglets caused by *E.coli* and Characterized by oedema of face, subcutis, encephalomalacia.

Etiology

- *E. coli* – Through faecal are route reaches in intestines and localizes through pili mediated attachment.
- Enterotoxins produced, damage to blood vessels.

- Oedema at subunits, face, colon, brain etc.
- Hemorrhagic gastroenteritis.

Clinical Manifestations

- Diarrhoea, melena.
- Fever, Oedema of face, eyelid, sub cutis.
- Death.

Macroscopic features

- Hemorrhagic gastroenteritis.
- Encephalomalacia.
- Oedema of colon, brain, stomach, small intestines.

Microscopic features

- Oedema in intestines.
- Hemorrhagic gastroenteritis.
- Encephalomalacia, hemorrhage in brain.
- Endocardial hemorrhage.

Diagnosis

- Symptoms and lesions.
- Isolation of bacteria.

3

Pathology of Chlamydial Diseases

Chlamydiosis

Chlamydiosis is an infectious disease of animals caused by Chlamydia sp. and characterized by encephalitis, polyarthritis and pneumonia in calves and abortions in cows and sheep.

Etiology

- *Chlamydia psittacii*

Pathogenesis

Chlamydial infection spreads through inhalation of contaminated dust from infected birds. Organism multiplies in lungs and through blood it spreads to liver, spleen, kidneys, brain, joints and placenta to cause pathology.

Characteristic symptoms

Calves

- Fever, dyspnoea
- Nasal discharge, hypersalivation
- Swelling of joints

Cows and Sheep

- Abortion at 7-9th month of gestation
- Subcutaneous oedema in foetus

Macroscopic features

Calves

- Serofibrinous peritonitis
- Enlargement of spleen

- Congestion of brain and spinal cord
- Oedema of synovial tissues
- Congestion and consolidation of lungs

Cows and Sheep

- Abortion
- Subcutaneous oedema in foetus
- Enlargement of lymph nodes, spleen
- Fibrino purulent exudate in placenta

Microscopic features

- Lobular pneumonia
- Congestion of brain and spinal cord
- Fibrinous exudate in synovial fluid
- Fibrino-purulent placentitis
- Bronchopneumonia
- Epithelization of alveolar cells

Diagnosis

- Symptoms and lesions
- Detection of antigen/antibody using ELISA
- Demonstration of chlamydial organism in synovial fluid, foetal stomach contents and lung tissue using special stains and immunoperoxidase techniques.
- Demonstration of chlamydial inclusions in tissue sections/impression smears.

4

Pathology of Rickettsial Diseases

Anaplasmosis

Anaplasmosis is an infectious disease of animals caused by a rickettsia and characterized by icterus, enlargement of spleen, pale tissues, thin watery blood and petechiae over serous membranes (Fig.4.1).

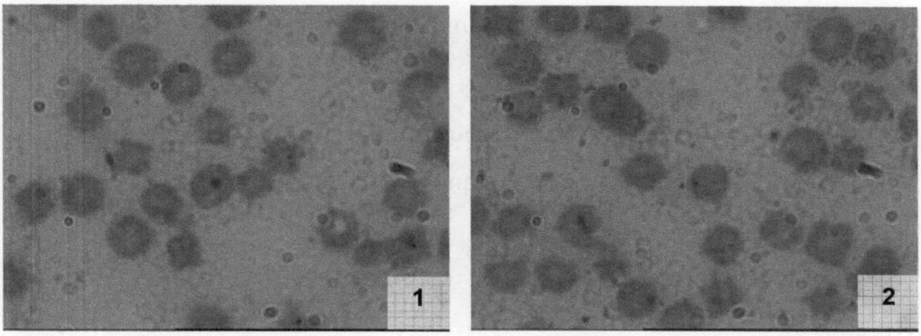

Fig. 4.1: Anaplasmosis in cattle- (1) Anaplasma centrale and (2) Anaplasma marginale infection.

Etiology

- *Anaplasma centrate*
- *A. marginale*
- *A. ovis*

Pathogenesis

The disease is transmitted through bite of tick (Boophilus), biting flies (Tabanus) and also in some cases due to mosquitoes. It is intra cellular organism and multiplies inside the erythrocytes by binary fission. The infected erythrocytes are engulfed by the cells of reticuloendothelial system (spleen, bone marrow). The process of erythrophagocytosis cause extra vascular haemolysis leading to anemia. It also causes autoimmune reaction leading to lysis of erythrocytes.

Characteristic symptoms

- High fever(105-107°F)
- Anemia
- Icterus

Macroscopic features

- Anemia, icterus
- Enlarged and yellow liver
- Petechiae on epicardium
- Enlargement of spleen
- Catarrhal exudate in intestines
- Gall bladder distended with granular bile.

Microscopic features

- Presence of organism in erythrocytes
- Haemorrhage in liver, kidneys and myocardium
- Necrosis in kidneys
- Haemosiderosis in spleen.

Diagnosis

- Demonstration of organism in blood smear
- Symptoms and lesions
- Immunodiagnostic tests for demonstration of antigen /antibody
- ELISA

Q – Fever

Q – Fever is an infectious disease of animals caused by rickettsia and characterized by fever, muscle and joint pain, diarrhea and respiratory distress. It is a zoonotic disease.

Etiology

- *Coxiella burnetti.*

Pathogenesis

- Mode of transmission is inhalation, contact.
- Incubation period 9-40 days.
- Through inhalation it causes flu like symptoms of fever, nasal discharge, body pain and respiratory distress.

Clinical Manifestations

- Fever, nasal discharge, nausea, diarrhoea.
- Muscle pain, joint Pain.
- Icterus, abortions.

Macroscopic features

- Rhinitis, pneumonia.
- Liver enlargement.
- Endocarditis.

Microscopic features

- Vasculitis.
- Endocarditis, myocarditis.
- Necrosis in liver.
- *Pneumonia.*
- Enteritis.

Diagnosis

- Symptoms & lesions.
- Detection of antigen and/or antibodies in blood/serum.

Ehrlichiosis

Ehrlichiosis in tick borne rickettsial disease of animals particularly dogs caused by *Ehrlichia* spp and Characterized by fever, vasculitis, lymphadenopathy, retinal hemorrhage and death.

Etiology

- *Ehrlichia canis.*
- Rickettsia, Tick borne.

Pathogenesis

- Transmitted through bite of tick, blood transfusions.
- Reaches in bone marrow, lymph nodes nervous system, eyes etc.
- Vaculitis in different organs.

Clinical Manifestations

- Fever, Petechiae on mucous membrane and skin.
- Bleeding disorder, lymphadenopathy.
- Oedema on lower parts of body.
- Polyuria, Polydipsia, dyspnea.
- Retinal hemorrhage, uveitis.

Macroscopic features

- Enlargement of lymph nodes.
- Retinal hemorrhage.
- Hemorrhage on vital organs of body – liver, Kidney, heart, lung, spleen.

Microscopic features

- Vasculitis.
- Hemorrhage in liver, Kidney, Spleen, lymph nodes.
- Blood examination – Pancytopenia.

Diagnosis

- Symptoms and lesions.
- Demonstration of rickettsia in blood cells during blood smear examination.

5

Pathology of Mycoplasmal Diseases

Contagious Bovine Pleuropneumonia (CBPP)

Contagious bovine pleuropneumonia (CBPP) is an infectious disease of cattle caused by *Mycoplasma* sp. and characterized by cuprous pneumonia, pleurisy and dilation of lymph vessels (Fig.5.1).

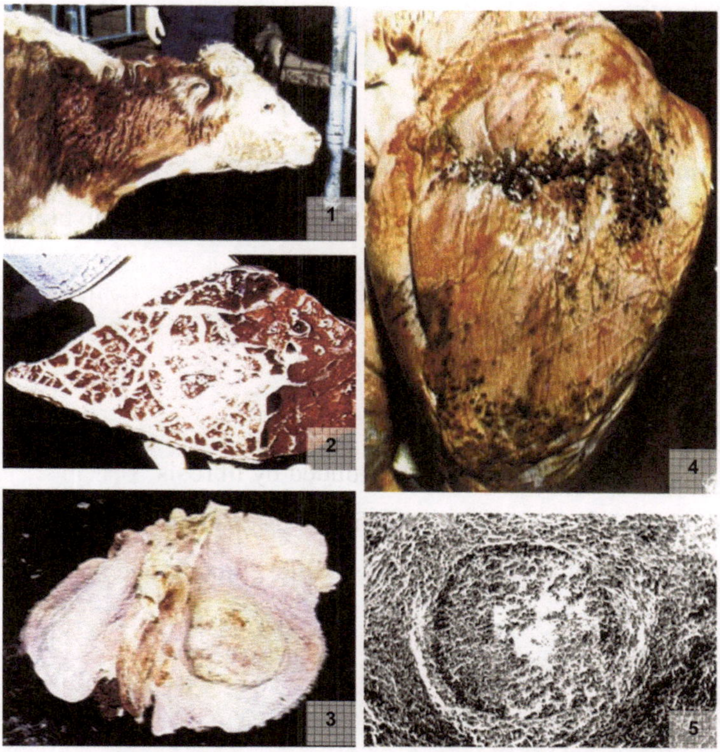

Fig.5.1: Contagious bovine pleuropneumonia (CBPP)- (1) Respiratory distress in cow, (2) Thickening of alveolar septa, (3) Presence of cheesy material in lung, (4) Petechial haemorrhages in pericardium and (5) Lymphofollicular reaction in mammary gland.

Etiology

- *Mycoplasma mycoides*

Pathogenesis

The infection spreads through inhalation of droplets from infected animals. The recovered animals act as source of infection at least for a period of 3 years. After entering through respiratory tract the organism reaches to bronchioles. It may remain in retropharyngeal gland from where it may spread in whole body. The organism from bronchioles enter into interlobular septa and causes inflammation followed by edema which causes dilation and subsequent thrombosis of lymph and blood vessels prior to development of pneumonic lesions. Death occurs due to anoxia and toxaemia.

Characteristic symptoms

- Fever (104-106°F)
- Dyspnoea
- Nasal discharge

Macroscopic features

- Congestion and consolidation of lungs with fibrinous adhesions in pleura
- Serofibrinous exudate in thoracic cavity
- Dilation of lymph vessels in lungs
- Marbled appearance on cut surfaces of lungs.

Microscopic features

- Thrombosis, ischemia and necrosis surrounded by fibrosis
- Thickening of alveolar septa due to serofibrinous exudate
- Congestion and consolidation of lung due to thickening of outer alveolar septa
- Serofibrinous pericarditis.

Diagnosis

- Symptoms and lesions
- Isolation of mycoplasma, nipple shaped colony on media
- Immunodiagnostic tests for demonstration of antigen / antibody using ELISA

- Demonstration of organisms in tissue sections using immunoperoxidase technique

Contagious Caprine Pleuropenumonia (CCPP)

Contagious caprine pleuropenumonia (CCPP) is an infectious disease of goats caused by *Mycoplasma* sp. and characterized by catarrh of upper respiratory tract, unilateral or bilateral pleuropneumonia, pleurisy, pericarditis and polyathritis (Fig.5.2).

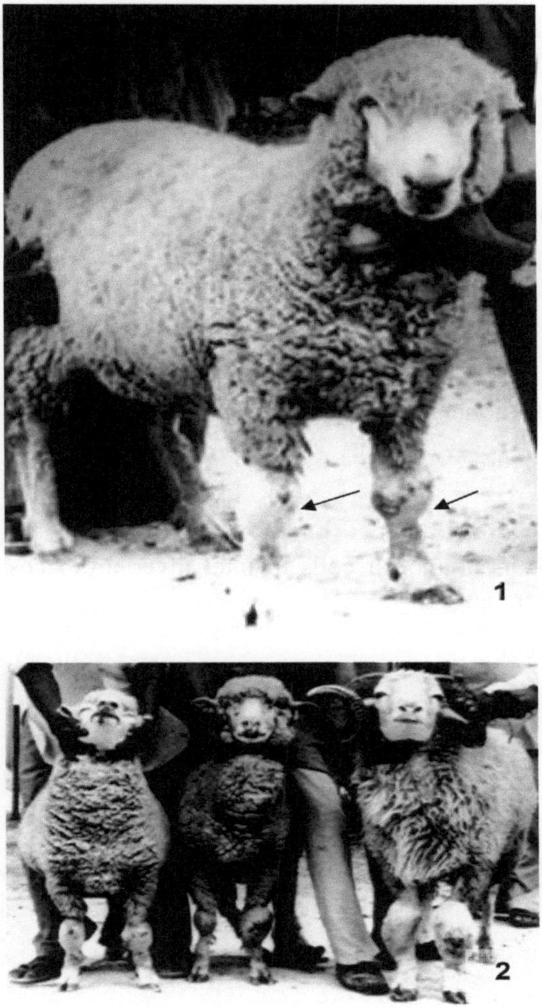

Fig. 5.2: Polyarthritis in sheep- (1&2) Swelling of knee joint in sheep.

Etiology

- *Mycoplasma mycoides*

Pathogenesis

The disease is readily spread by inhalation but organism does not survive for long period out side the animal body and its pathogenesis is just like CBPP.

Characteristic symptoms

- Fever (103-106°F)
- Dyspnoea
- Nasal discharge

Macroscopic features

- Rhinitis and catarrh of upper respiratory tract
- Congestion and consolidation of lungs
- Pleurisy with gelatinous exudate
- Fibrinous pericarditis
- Oedema and congestion of bronchial and mediastinal lymph nodes.
- Adhesions of lungs with pleura

Microscopic features

- Congestion, infiltration of mononuclear cells in inter alveolar spaces; formation of lymphoid aggregates
- Deposition of fibrin in alveoli
- Fibrinous pericarditis
- Oedema and congestion in lymph nodes.

Diagnosis

- Symptoms and lesions
- Isolation of mycoplasma, nipple shaped colony on media
- Immunodiagnostic tests for demonstration of antigen /antibody
- ELISA

- Demonstration of organisms in tissue sections using immunoperoxidase technique

Mycoplasmal Abortion

Mycoplasmosis specially abortions in cattle due to mycoplasma is a disease of adult cattle caused by several species of *Mycoplasma* sp. and characterized by abortions in pregnant animals, mastitis and pneumonia and polyarthritis in foetus.

Etiology

- *Mycoplasma mycoides*
- *M. bovigenitalium*

Pathogenesis

Pathogenesis is not exactly known. However, this organism is considered to be non-pathogenic for animals. But in a state of immunosuppression, it may cause illness as opportunistic pathogen.

Characteristic Symptoms

- Abortion in cattle
- Mucous discharge from vagina
- Hard swelling of udder in mastitis

Macroscopic features

- Abortion in cattle
- Bronchopneumonia in foetus
- Oedema of placenta

Microscopic features

- Lymphoid infiltration and aggregation of lymphocytes in placenta, uterus and in mammary gland.
- Lymphofollicular reaction in lungs and liver in foetus.

Diagnosis

- Serological examination-detection of antibody or antigen
- Isolation of mycoplasma using ELISA

- Demonstration of organism in tissue sections using immunoperoxidase technique

Porcine enzootic pneumonia

Porcine enzootic pneumonia is an infectious disease of pigs caused by *Mycoplasma hyopneumoniae* and characterized by catarrh of upper respiratory tract, unilateral or bilateral pneumonia.

Etiology

- *Mycoplasma hyopneumoniae*.

Pathogen is

- Transmission though direct contact.
- Incubation period 2-6 weeks.
- Piglets of more than 6 weeks of age are mainly affected.
- Organism attaches to the cilia in the trachea, bronchi.
- Clumping and loss of cilia and excessive production of mucous.
- Lead to immunosuppression and may attract PRPS, PCV2, *P. multocida, B. bronchiseptica* infection.

Clinical Manifestations

- Fever (103-106° F), Dyspnoea, nasal discharge.
- Reduced growth rate and feed efficiency.
- Coughing, prostration and death.

Macroscopic features

- Rhinitis and catarrh of upper respiratory pact.
- Pneumonia, Pleurisy with gelatinous exudate.
- Fibrinous pericarditis.
- Adhesions of lungs with pleura.
- Swollen and congested lymph nodes.

Microscopic features

- Congestion, infiltration of mononuclear cells in lungs at inter alveolar spaces.
- Lymphofollicular reaction
- Fibrinous pericarditis.
- Oedema and congestion of lymph nodes.

Diagnosis

- Symptoms and lesions.
- Isolation of mycoplasma.
- Demonstration of organism in tissues using immunohistochemical techniques.

6

Pathology of Spirochaetal Diseases

Leptospirosis

Leptospirosis is an infectious disease of animals caused by spirocheate *Leptospria* sp. and characterized by widespread haemorrhage in visceral organs, nephritis, icterus, hepatitis and anemia (Fig.6.1).

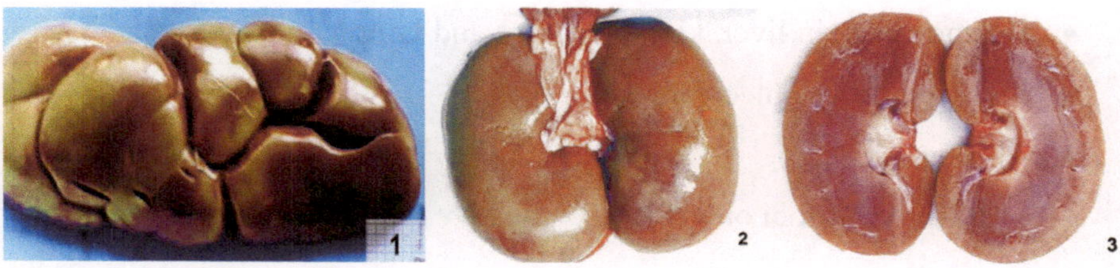

Fig. 6.1: Leptospirosis in animals- **(1)** Petechial haemorrhage and necrosis on kidney of cattle and **(2 & 3)** dogs.

Etiology

- *Leptospira ictehaemorrhagae*
- *L. pomona*

Pathogenesis

The organism is transmitted through direct contact with urine of infected animals or ingestion of urine contaminated feed or water. It can also be transmitted through aborted fetuses and infected uterine discharges. The organism enters through abraded skin and mucous membrane and reaches in blood and multiplies rapidly in blood producing septicemia and high rise in body temperature. Thereafter the organism localizes in the kidneys leading to acute or chronic nephritis. In kidneys, it multiplies in proximal convoluted tubules (PCT) and is excreted in urine which acts as source of infection.

Characteristic symptoms

- High fever(105-107°F)
- Anemia
- Icterus
- Abortion, mastitis
- Haemoglobinuria

Macroscopic features

- Anemia, icterus
- Haemoglobinuria
- Blood mixed milk
- Haemorrhage in liver, kidneys, lungs and lymph nodes
- Enlargement of spleen and kidneys
- Abortion
- Grayish white foci on visceral organs.

Microscopic features

- Necrosis and hyperplasia of kupffer's cells in liver
- Necrosis of tubular epithelium and formation hyaline in tubules of kidneys along with lymphocytic infiltration
- Haemosiderosis in spleen
- Encephalitis.

Diagnosis

- Symptoms and lesions
- Demonstrations of leptospira in urine samples under dark field microscopy
- Isolation of leptospira
- Immunodiagnostic tests for demonstration of antigen /antibody
- ELISA
- Demonstration of organism in tissue sections using special stains

7

Pathology of Prion Diseases

Spongiform encephalopathy

Spongiform encephalopathy is an infectious disease of animals caused by prion proteins and characterized by presence of vacuoles in brain.

Etiology

- Prion proteins
- Sheep – Scrapie or Ovine spongiform encephalopathy
- Cattle - Bovine spongiform encephalopathy (Mad cow disease)
- Feline encephalopathy

Pathogenesis

Scrapie is also known as ovine spongiform encephalopathy. The principle means of transmission of disease is from infected mother to their lambs early in life; placental transmission has also been reported. The incubation period of disease is very long (2-5 year). The clinical form is restricted in adults. The prion proteins (PrP) occur normally in the central nervous system of all domestic animals and man bounded with neuronal surface. Animal susceptible to prion disease have a gene (PrP gene) which encodes for normal "Prion protein (PrP)" or "cellular prion protein (PrPc). In scrapie prion protein (PrPsc)/ scrapie associated fibril protein (SAI) is generated which are resistant for protease digestion. Accumulation of PrPsc in neural tissues appears to be the cause of the pathology in prion disease. When prion protein contaminated meat and bone meal are fed to the cattle as part of their concentration, the agent (prion) got introduced into cattle. Prion protein (PrP) on reaching brain slowly and progressively converted into and abnormal form (PrP sc) and this abnormal protein causes development of lesions including vacuolation in nerve cells.

Characteristic symptoms

- No characteristic symptom
- Circling movements of animal
- Itching in skin in sheep suffering from scrapie

Macroscopic features

- No gross lesion

Microscopic features

- Presence of large vacuoles in the cytoplasm of neurons in medulla oblongata, midbrain and spinal cord
- Brain looks like sponge
- Inflammatory changes like infiltration of cells, congestion, haemorrhages are absent
- Occasionally accumulation of lymphocytes in Vircho-Robin spaces.

Diagnosis

- History of case
- Symptoms and lesions
- Vacuoles in neurons
- Histopathological examination of brain tissue

8

Pathology of Fungal Diseases

Ringworm

Ringworm is a fungal disease of skin affecting animals characterized by popular skin lesions in circular form discharging serus exudate.

Etiology

- *Microsporum canis*- dogs
- *M. gypseum*- dogs, horse, pig
- *Trichophyton verrucosum*- bovines
- *T. equinum*- horses

Pathogenesis

The fungi enter in skin through abrasion and the hyphae appear in stratum corneum after germination and invade the hair follicles. The hyphae growth and spore formation in stratum corneum leads to hyperkeratosis and the fungus spreads centrifugally from the point of primary invasion leading to ring shaped lesion (Fig.8.1).

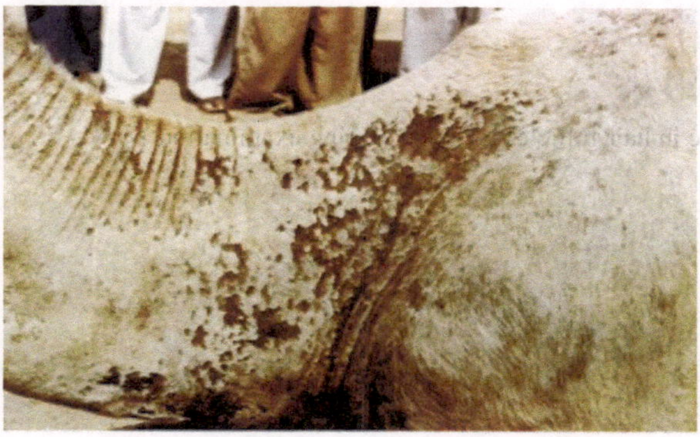

Fig. 8.1: Ringworm in camel

Characteristics Symptoms

- Ring shaped lesions on skin
- Serum's discharge from lesions
- Hyperkeratosis, severe itching
- Loss of hairs

Macroscopic features

- Ring shaped lesions on skin of face, around eyes, neck and shoulder
- Loss of hairs with raised, dry, crusty and grayish white masses
- Hyperkeratosis

Microscopic features

- Presence of hyphae in hair follicles
- Hyperkeratosis of skin

Diagnosis

- Symptoms and lesions
- Demonstration of hyphae in hair follicles/skin scrapings (Fig.8 2)

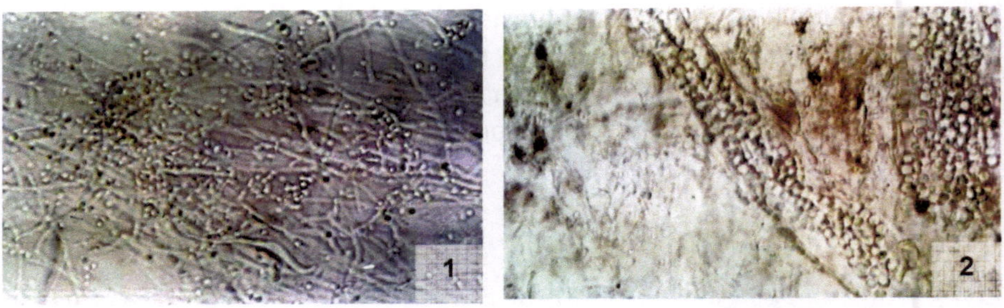

Fig. 8.2: (1&2) Presence of hyphae in hair follicles on skin scraping examination.

- Demonstration of fungus in lesions using Wood's lamp
- Isolation of fungus in SDA media

Candidiasis

Candidiasis is a fungal disease of animals caused by *Candida albicans* and characterized by a variety of manifestations including mastitis, chronic pneumonia, vaginal discharges, abortion and oesophagitis.

Etiology

- *Candida albicans*
- Yeast like cells, oval, 3.5-5.5μ size

Pathogenesis

The fungus may enter through inhalation, ingestion or through abraded mucous membrane. It causes rumenitis and oesophagitis in calves with chronic lesions. It is thought to occur as a result of heavy antibacterial therapy and may cause mastitis, pneumonia and/or abortion.

Characteristic Symptoms

- Cutaneous granulomatous lesions in dogs and cats
- Difficulty in ingestion
- Hard udder
- Vaginal discharges/abortion

Macroscopic features

- Chronic pneumonic lesions- nodules in lungs
- Oesophagitis
- Cutaneous nodular lesions
- Rumenitis

Microscopic features

- In tissue sections presence of candida as round or oval budding cells with pseudomycelia.
- Chronic granulomatous lesions

Diagnosis

- Symptoms and lesions
- Demonstration of candida in skin scrapings or lesions
- Isolation of fungus

Rhinosporidiosis

Rhinosporidiosis is a fungal disease of cattle and buffaloes caused by *Rhinosporidium* sp. and characterized by polypoid growth on nasal mucosa and dyspnea (Fig.8.3).

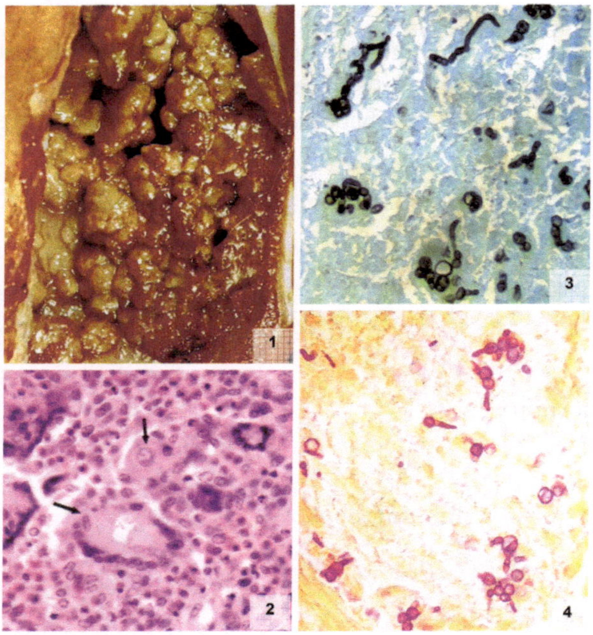

Fig. 8.3: Rhinosporidiosis- (1) Polypoid growth in nasal cavity, (2) Granulomatous inflammation around fungus and (3&4) Demonstration of fungal conidia and hyphae in tissue sections.

Etiology

- *Rhinosporidum seeberi*

Pathogenesis

Fungus enters through abraded skin/mucous membrane and causes hyperplasia of stratum spinosum.

Characteristic Symptoms

- Dyspnoea
- Sneezing
- Mucopurulent nasal discharge

Macroscopic features

- Nasal polyps from small size to several centimeters in diameter filling whole nasal cavity.
- Papular lesions on conjunctival sac, ears and vagina.

Microscopic features

- Fibromyxomatous lesion with numerous blood vessels
- Presence of white specks consists of sporangia filled with endospores.

Diagnosis

- Symptoms and lesions
- Microscopic examination of nasal polyps
- Demonstration of causative fungi in tissue sections using special stains

Aspergillosis

Aspergillosis is a fungal disease of animals characterized by granulomatous pulmonary lesions, abortion and lobar pneumonia in foetus.

Etiology

- *Aspergillus fumigatus* (Fig.8.4)

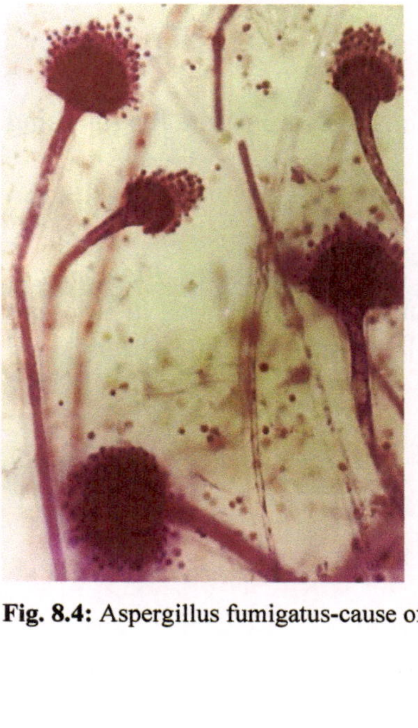

Fig. 8.4: Aspergillus fumigatus-cause of aspergillosis.

- Dark green conidia

Pathogenesis

Aspergillus enters in body through mouldy grains or inhalation. In lungs fungi causes chronic granuloma formation leading to nodules with caseation and fibrosis.

Characteristic Symptoms

- Nasal discharge
- Sneezing/coughing
- Abortion in ewes

Macroscopic features

- Tubercle like granulomatous lesions in lungs
- Abortion in ewes and cattle
- Lobar pneumonia in aborted foetus

Microscopic features

- Granulomatous lesions in lungs
- Fungus can be demonstrated in lesions

Diagnosis

- Symptoms and lesions
- Microscopic examination of tissue sections to demonstrate fungus using special stain

Blastomycosis

Blastomycosis is a systemic fungal disease of animals caused by *Blastomyces dermatitidis* and characterized by chronic granulomatous lesions in skin and other internal organs including lymph nodes, liver, spleen, kidneys, lungs and intestines (Fig.8.5).

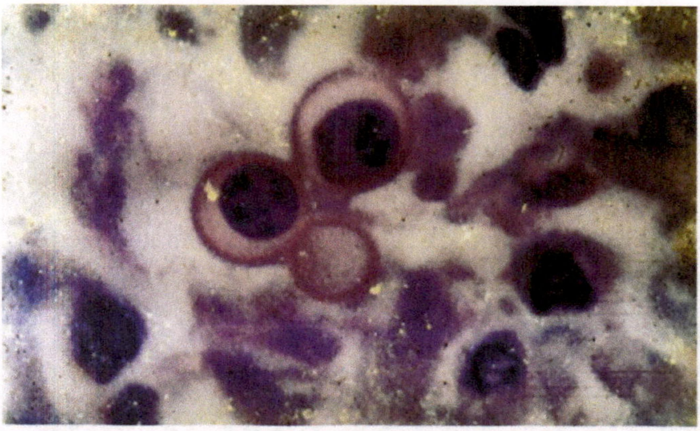

Fig. 8.5: Blastomycosis- Blastomyces dermatitidis in tissue section of lung covered by macrophages and lymphocytes.

Etiology

- *Blastomyces dermatitidis*
- Yeast like bodies in tissues

Pathogenesis

Organism causes chronic granulomatous inflammation of skin and internal organs.

Characteristic Symptoms

- Nodules on skin
- Debilitating condition of animal
- Lameness
- Swelling and hardness of superficial lymph nodes

Macroscopic features

- Presence of nodules on skin, lymph nodes, lungs, kidneys and liver
- Papule or pustule on skin

Microscopic features

- Presence of yeast like bodies in chronic granulomatous lesions

Diagnosis

- Symptoms and lesions
- Identification of fungus in tissue sections using special stains

Coccidioidomycosis

Coccidioidomycosis is a systemic fungal disease of animals characterized by granulomatous lesions in lymph nodes and lungs (Fig.8.6).

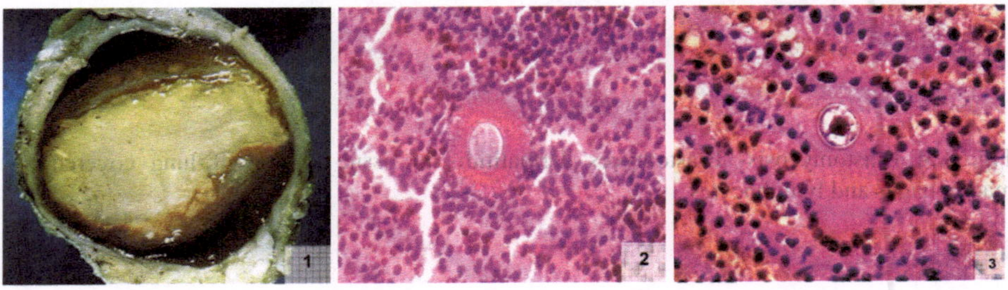

Fig. 8.6: Coccidioidomycosis- (1) Chronic suppurative lymphadenitis, (2) Presence of Coccidioides immitis in tissue section with sulfur club like structures and (3) Coccidioides immitis within a giant.

Etiology

- *Coccidioides immitis*
- Spherical bodies- sporangia

Pathogenesis

Desert rodents normally inhabit the fungus and excrete large number of spherules through faeces in soil, which germinate and multiply in soil after rain. When the ground dries, large number of arthroconidia are produced and released in air. Animals get infection through air during grazing that produces lesions in lungs and lymph nodes.

Characteristic Symptoms

- Nasal discharge
- Sneezing or coughing
- Nodular lesions on skin

Macroscopic features

- Nodular lesions in lungs and lymph nodes

- Thick, yellow, gelatinous pus in lesion
- Abscess wall shows granulation tissue

Microscopic features

- Granulomatous lesions in mediastinal, bronchial, submaxillary, retropharyngeal and mesenteric lymph nodes
- Granulomatous lesions in lungs

Diagnosis

- Symptoms and lesions
- Demonstration of fungus in tissue sections using special stains

Cryptococcosis

Cryptococcosis is a systemic fungal disease of animals characterized by nervous disorders including encephalitis, meningitis and presence of granuloma in eyes, sinuses and nasal septum.

Etiology

- *Cryptococcus neoformans*
- Spherical or ovoid shape, thick walled, single or budding, 3-8 μm diameter.

Pathogenesis

The organism is normally found in soil. Cryptococcosis occurs in animals through inhalation or implantation. In cows, it can enter through teat canal. It slowly reaches to the central nervous system due to its tropism to nervous tissue. Presence of capsule saves the organism from phagocytosis.

Characteristic Symptoms

- Nervous signs including in coordination of movements, staggering gait.
- Sneezing or coughing

Macroscopic features

- Encephalitis
- Pneumonia
- Granuloma in nasal mucosa and meninges

- Granulomatous lesions in eyes, sinuses and nasal septum
- Mastitis
- Enlargement of lymph nodes

Microscopic features

- Encephalitis and meningitis
- Pleocytosis
- Granulomatous lesions in lymph nodes
- Presence of cryptococcus in tissue sections

Diagnosis

- Symptoms and lesions
- Demonstration of fungus in tissue sections using special stains
- Isolation of fungus

Histoplasmosis

Histoplasmosis is a systemic fungal disease of animals characterized by chronic pneumonia, spleenomegaly, hepatomegaly, leucopenia and ulcers in intestines.

Etiology

- *Histoplasma capsulatum*
- Intracellular, chlamydocondia- round, thick walled structure 7-15 μ diameter.

Pathogenesis

Air borne infection of histoplasma reaches to the lungs where it is phagccytosed by the reticuloendothelial cells that disseminate the infection in different organs/tissues.

Characteristic Symptoms

- Leucopenia
- Diarrhoea
- Anemia

- Sneezing / coughing
- Pyrexia
- Dyspnoea
- Emaciation
- Enlarged abdomen

Macroscopic features

- Spleenomegaly
- Hepatomegaly
- Ulcers in intestines
- Lymphadenopathy
- Ascites

Microscopic features

- Organism packed in macrophages
- Granulomatous lesions in lungs, liver, spleen and lymph nodes

Diagnosis

- Symptoms and lesions
- Demonstration of fungus in macrophages in tissue sections using special stains
- Isolation of fungus

Mucous Mycosis

Mucous mycosis is caused by *Absidia* sp. and characterized by chronic inflammation of lymph nodes, lung, uterus and placenta (Fig. 8.7).

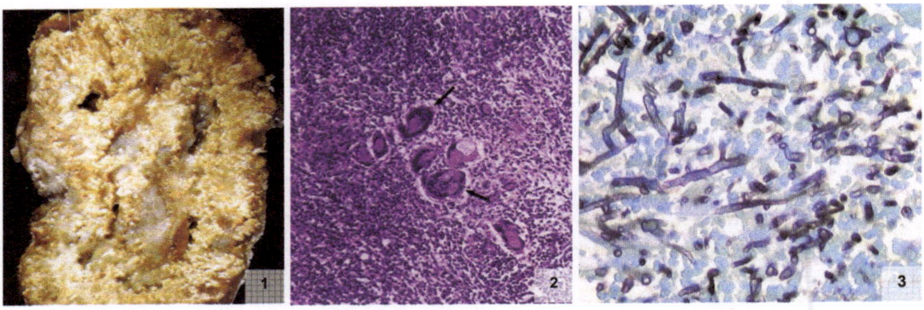

Fig. 8.7: Mucormycosis in animals- (1) Granulomatous lesions in mediastinal lymph node, (2) Presence of several giant cells (arrow) in the inflammation and (3) Mycelium of the fungus in tissue (Gomori's Stain).

Etiology

- *Absidia corymbifera*

Pathogenesis

Not clear

Characteristic Symptoms

- Abortion
- Chronic wasting- progressive weakness

Macroscopic features

- Granulomatous lesions in lungs, lymph nodes placenta, uterus
- Thick, hard, tubercle like nodules
- Cheesy exudate with calcification
- Reddish gray exudate with pus flukes in interplacentome space.

Microscopic features

- Granulomatous lesions in lungs, lymph nodes
- Infiltration of neutrophils, macrophages, lymphocytes, eosinophils, giant cells.
- Calcification of centrally caseative necrosed area.

Diagnosis

- Symptoms and lesions
- Demonstration of fungus in tissues
- Isolation of fungus.

Degnala Disease

Degnala disease is a non-infectious disease of animals caused by mycotoxins and characterized by dry gangrene on extremities such as tip of ear, tail and hooves with sloughing of hooves (Fig.8.8).

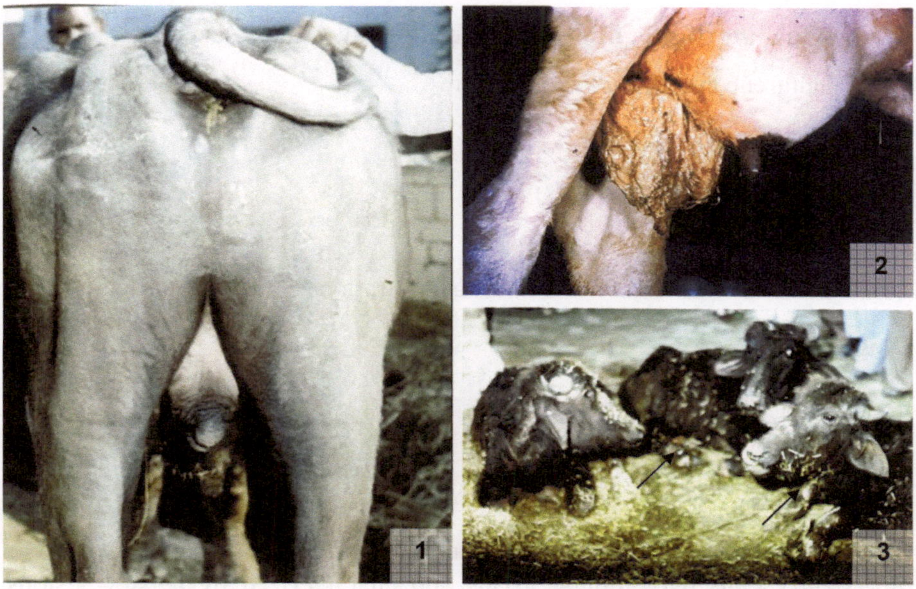

Fig. 8.8: Degnala disease in animals- (1) Presence of dry gangrene on tip of serotum (2) Sloughing of skin from teats/udder due to gangrene and (3) Sloughing of hooves (arrow).

Etiology

- *Fusarium tricinctum*
- Mycotoxins of fungus
- Paddy straw infested with fungus is source of mycotoxin.

Pathogenesis

Ingestion of mycotoxin in feed causes vasoconstriction leading to infarction, necrosis at extremities. Saprophytes invade and form dry gangrene.

Characteristic Symptoms

- Dry gangrene on tail, ear, scrotum and hooves
- Sloughing of skin
- Lameness

Macroscopic features

- Sloughing of skin from hooves leaving raw wound surface
- Gangrene at tail, ears and scrotum

Microscopic features

- Loss of architectural details
- Necrosis
- Oedema with slight mononuclear infiltration

Diagnosis

- Symptoms and lesions
- Detection of toxin in feed

Aflatoxicosis

Aflatoxicosis is a toxic condition of animals widely prevalent in all parts of the country caused by fungal toxins and characterized by hepatic lesions, immunosuppression and cancer.

Etiology

- Fungal toxins of *Aspergillus flavus* and *Penicillium puberlum* and several other fungi.
- Aflatoxin B1, B2, G1, G2, M1, M2.

Pathogenesis

After ingestion aflatoxin, under goes biotransformation into highly reactive metabolites which binds with nucleic acids and reduce protein synthesis and causes immunosuppression. These metabolic alterations cause enlargement of liver, spleen and kidneys and atrophy of lymphoid organs.

Characteristic symptoms

- Enlargement of abdomen
- Anemia
- Immunosuppression
- Decreased production
- Retarded growth of animals

Macroscopic features

- Enlargement of liver
- Necrotic foci in liver.
- Congestion and hemorrhage in liver.
- Tumourous nodules in liver.
- Atrophy of spleen.
- Hemorrhage in muscles.

Microscopic features

- Necrosis in hepatic parenchyma.
- Proliferation of bile duct epithelium.
- Fibrosis in liver.
- Hemorrhage in muscles and myocardium.

Diagnosis

- Symptoms and lesions
- Detection of toxins in feed/tissues of affected animals using TLC or flurotoxinometer.
- Immunodiagnostic tests for detection of aflatoxins in feed and tissues.
- ELISA
- DIA

Ochratoxicosis

Ochratoxicosis is a toxic condition of animals caused by a fungal toxin and characterized by nephrosis, pale bone marrow and hemorrhage in intestines.

Etiology

- Ochratoxins produced by *Aspergillus ochraceous* and several other species of *Aspergillus* and *Penicillium* sp.

Pathogenesis

Ochratoxin is found in maize and in most of the small grains contaminated with moulds. It inhibits protein synthesis, produces acute proximal tubular epithelial necrosis in kidneys and inhibits normal renal uric acid excretion.

Characteristic symptoms

- Anemia
- Increased clotting time
- Loss of pigmentation

Macroscopic features

- Enlargement of kidneys
- Deposition of urates on kidneys
- Haemorrhage in kidneys
- Haemorrhage in duodenum.
- Anemia
- Pale bone marrow.
- Atrophy of lymphoid organs
- Ascites

Microscopic features

- Nephrosis, deposition of urates.
- Infiltration of neutrophils and fibrosis.
- Haemorrhage in intestinal wall.
- Lymphoid depletion in spleen.

Diagnosis

- Symptoms and lesions
- Detection of ochratoxin in feed/tissues using TLC/HPLC methods.
- Immunodiagnostic tests for detection of toxins in feed
- ELISA
- DIA

Trichothecene toxicity

Trichothecene toxicosis occurs in animals as a result of feeding of contaminated feed caused by mycotoxin trichothecene and characterized by gastroenteritis, immunosuppression and death.

Etiology

- Mycotoxins – Trichothecene having following components:
  - Deoxynivalenol (DON) or Vomitoxin
  - T- 2 toxin
  - Diacetoxyscirpenol (DAS).
  - Satratoxin, roridin, verrucarin.
- Of these, DON is most common contaminant of corn, wheat and other grains.
- T -2 toxin and DAS are sporadic.
- Produced by fungus-*Fusarium* spp, *Trichothecium* spp, *Myrothecium* Spp, and *Cephalosporium* Spp.

Pathogenesis

- Enters in body through ingestion.
- Absorbed through intestine, causing damage to intestinal epithelial cells.
- Inhibits protein synthesis.
- Leads to gastroenteritis, immunosuppression.

Clinical Manifestation

- Diarrhoea, Melena
- Stomatitis.

- Hyperkeratosis.
- Ulceration on skin.

Macroscopic feathers

- Stomatitis, ulcers in oesophagus.
- Necrosis of G.I. tract mucosa.
- Ulcers on Skin.
- Hyperkeratosis.

Microscopic features

- Gastroenteritis, necrosis of epithelium of intestines.
- Hyperkeratosis
- Lymphoid depletion.
- Lymphopenia, Pancytopenia.

Diagnosis

- Symptoms and lesions.
- Detection of toxins in feed, tissue, blood.

Ergotoxicois /Ergotism

Ergotism occurs in animals as a result of feeding of mycotoxins of fungus *Claviceps purprea* and characterized by Fever, hyper salivation, lameness, and agalactia after parturition.

Etiology

- Ergot produced by *Claviceps purpurea* fungus in grains, seed heads.
- Alkaloid – Ergotamine, Ergonovine.
- More than 200 ppb – toxic.

Pathogenesis

- Causes vasoconstriction, gangrene at extremities.
- Stimulation of CNS followed by depression.
- Inhibit pituitary release of prolactin leads to failure of mammary development in late gestation.

- Agalactia.

Clinical Manifestations

- Fever, hyper salivation, lameness.
- Gangrene at extremities.
- Agalactia.

Macroscopic features

- Gangrene at extremities.
- Pale, anemic mucous membranes.
- Subcutaneous hemorrhages.

Microscopic features

- Necrosis, gangrene on Skin.
- Oedema, hemorrhage in skin and mucous membrane.
- Thrombosis.
- Necrosis of vascular endothelium.

Diagnosis

- Symptoms and lesions.
- Detection of ergot in feed, grains, hay.

9

Pathology of Parasitic Diseases

Trypanosomosis

Trypanosomosis is an infectious disease of animals caused by protozoan parasite and characterized by emaciation, enlargement of spleen and lymph nodes, petechiae on serous membranes, ulceration on tongue and gastric mucosa and gelatinous exudate in subcutaneous region.

Etiology

- *Trypanosoma evansi*

Pathogenesis

The disease is mainly transmitted through bite of flies like Tabanus, Stomoxys, Haematopota etc. The carrier animals remain as potential source of infection. The pathogenesis of disease is not completely known. After entering in mammalian host, trypanosomes multiply in blood stream by binary fission leading to parasitaenia. The parasites has variable surface glycoproteins which cause continuous exposure of immune system leading to hyperplasia of spleen and lymph nodes. In chronic cases, due to formation of antigen- antibody complexes glomerulonephritis and vasculitis is seen.

Characteristic symptoms

- High fever (105-107°F)
- Dyspnoea
- Paraplegia, emaciation
- Oedema in dependent parts of body
- Conjunctivitis, keratitis

Macroscopic features

- Emaciated carcass
- Enlargement of spleen and lymph nodes
- Gelatinous exudate in subcutaneous region
- Ulcerative keratitis
- Congestion of abomasum and intestines
- Petechiae on kidneys, liver and heart
- Ulcers in tongue and abomasum.

Microscopic features

- Presence of flagellate parasite in blood smear (Fig.9.1)

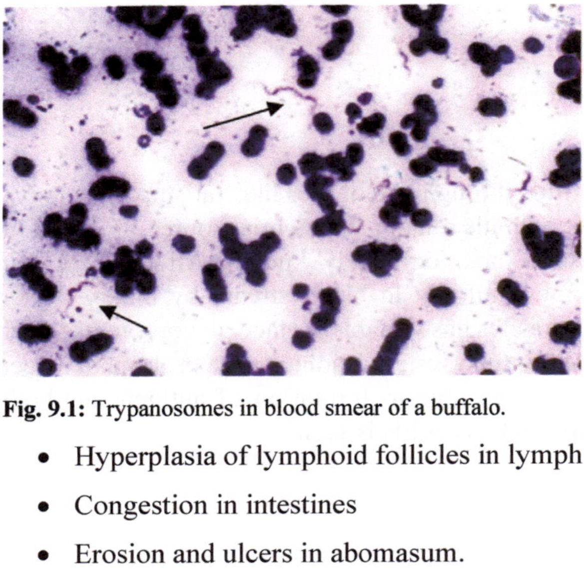

Fig. 9.1: Trypanosomes in blood smear of a buffalo.

- Hyperplasia of lymphoid follicles in lymph nodes and spleen
- Congestion in intestines
- Erosion and ulcers in abomasum.

Diagnosis

- Demonstration of protozoan parasite in blood smear
- Symptoms and lesions
- Immunodiagnostic tests for demonstration of antigen /antibody
- ELISA

Theileriosis

Theileriosis is an infectious disease of animals caused by protozoan parasite and characterized by enlargement of lymph nodes, pulmonary oedema, haemorrhage in kidneys and liver, ulcers in abomasum and catarrhal enteritis.

Etiology

- *Theileria annulata*

Pathogenesis

The parasite is transmitted through bite of ticks of genus Hyalomma. The disease can also be transmitted mechanically by inoculation of blood and tissue suspension made from spleen, lymph nodes and liver of infected animals. After entry the organism at sporozoit stage remains in blood circulation and enters in erythrocytes but they don't multiply. The multiplication occurs in lymphocytes where it forms schizonts. Infected lymphocytes are ruptured and schizonts are released and other lymphocytes are affected. Later some schizonts are differentiated unto merozoites. The rapidly multiplying schizonts are causing severe damage to lymphoid cells through their lysis.

Characteristic symptoms

- High fever (105-107°F)
- Anemia
- Enlargement of superficial lymph nodes

Macroscopic features

- Anemia
- Pulmonary oedema
- Enlargement of lymph nodes and spleen
- Erosions and ulcers in abomasum
- Haemorrhage in epicardium
- Catarrhal enteritis

Microscopic features

- Lymphoid depletion
- Presence of parasites in erythrocytes or its developmental stages in lymphocytes

- Perivascular lymphoid proliferation
- Congestion in intestines
- Proliferation of goblet cells.

Diagnosis

- Demonstration of protozoan parasite in blood smear/lymph node biopsy (Fig.9.2)

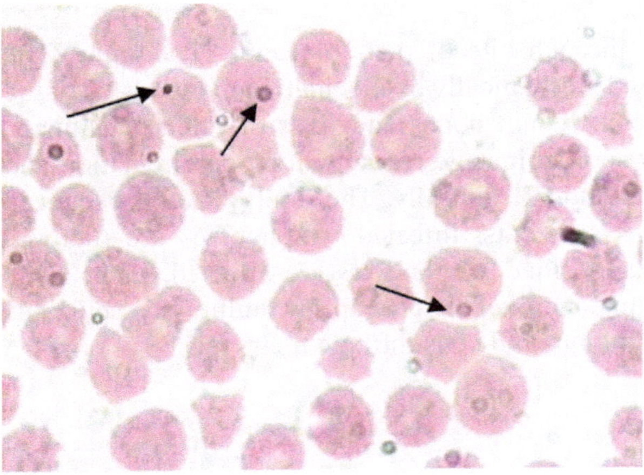

Fig. 9.2: Theileria sp. in erythrocytes of a cow.

- Symptoms and lesions
- Immunodiagnostic tests for demonstration of antigen /antibody
- ELISA

Babesiosis

Babesiosis is an infectious disease of animals caused by protozoan parasite and characterized by hemoglobinuria, anemia, petechiae and ecchymoses in serous membranes, icterus, pulmonary oedema and gastroenteritis.

Etiology

- *Babesia bigemina*
- *B. bovis*

Pathogenesis

The disease is transmitted from sick to healthy animal through ticks following trans ovarian route. The incubation period of disease is 5-10 days. After infection, the parasite multiplies in peripheral blood and there is intra-vascular haemolysis leading to hemoglobinuria. The infected erythrocytes liberate some enzymes which interact with the components of blood and leads to increased erythrocyte fragility, hypertensive shock and disseminated intra ocular coagulation.

Characteristic symptoms

- High fever (105-107°F)
- Anemia, icterus
- Hemoglobinuria

Macroscopic features

- Anemia, icterus
- Hemoglobinuria
- Enlargement of spleen and liver
- Oedema in lungs
- Petechiae and ecchymoses in kidneys, lungs, liver and spleen
- Congestion in gastrointestinal tract

Microscopic features

- Presence of pear shaped Babesia organism in erythrocytes
- Haemorrhage in liver, kidneys, lungs and spleen
- Haemosiderosis in spleen
- Necrosis of tubular epithelium in kidneys and presence of hyaline casts.

Diagnosis

- Demonstration of protozoan parasite in blood smear (Fig. 9.3)

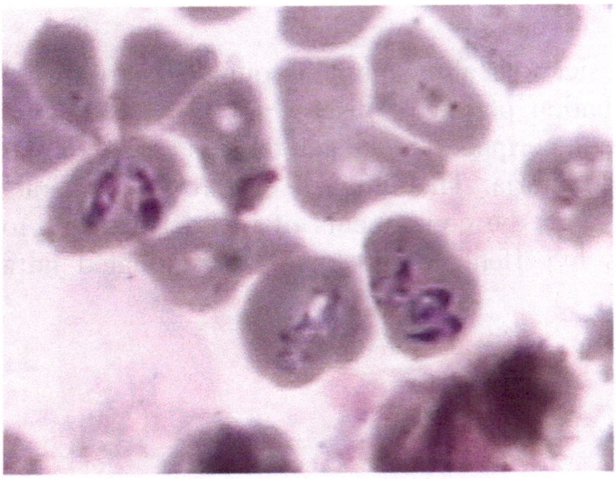

Fig. 9.3: Babesia bigemina in erythrocytes of a cow.

- Symptoms and lesions
- Immunodiagnostic tests for demonstration of antigen /antibod
- ELISA

Trichomoniasis

Trichomoniasis is a protozoan parasitic disease of animals caused by *Trichomonas* sp. characterized by abortion, vaginitis, metritis and balanitis in cattle and gastroenteritis in horses.

Etiology

- *Trichomonas foetus*- cattle
- *T. faecalis*- horses
- *T. suis*- swine
- *T. gallinae*- poultry

Pathogenesis

Following coitus, cow gets infection from bull that causes vaginitis, endometritis, placentitis, foetal infection and abortion in early gestation. Abortion followed by pyometra due to invasion of secondary bacterial infection.

Characteristic Symptoms

- Abortion
- Retention of placenta

- Sterility
- Pyometra

Macroscopic features

- Vaginitis
- Gastroenteritis in horses
- Metritis- Pyometra
- Abortion during 3-5 month of gestation
- Balanitis in bulls

Microscopic features

- Infilteration of neutrophils in uterus.
- Presence of trichomonads in tissue sections of uterus.

Diagnosis

- Symptoms and lesions
- Demonstration of trichomonads in prepuceal washing and vaginal discharges
- Demonstration of trichononades in uterine tissue sections

Toxoplasmosis

Toxoplasmosis is a protozoan parasitic disease of animals characterized by encephalitis, foetalization of lungs, ulcers in intestines, necrosis in liver and abortion.

Etiology

- *Toxoplasma gondii*
- Immunosuppression predisposes animals and reactivation of parasites to cause disease.

Pathogenesis

Transmission of parasite occurs through ingestion of contaminated meat or feed. The sporozoites penetrate intestinal wall and multiply. Thereafter, they reach to the other organs through blood stream. In brain it causes encephalitis; infection may also occur in foetus as congenital that leads to pneumonia, enterocolitis and skin lesions.

Characteristic Symptoms

- Convulsions
- Nasal discharge
- Nervous signs- staggering gait, incoordination in moments.

Macroscopic features

- Necrosis in brain and liver
- Nodules in lungs
- Ulcers in intestines
- Oedema in placenta

Microscopic features

- Lymphocytic infilteration in brain, pancreas, lungs and myocardium.
- Coaggulative necrosis in liver
- Fetalization of lung alveolar lung epithelium becomes cubcidal or columnar.
- Granulomatous inflammation in intestines.

Diagnosis

- Symptoms and lesions
- Serological examination- ELISA
- Demonstration of parasites

Coccidiosis

Coccidiosis is protozoan parasitic disease of animals characterized by gastroenteritis, hepatitis and typhlitis (Fig. 9.4).

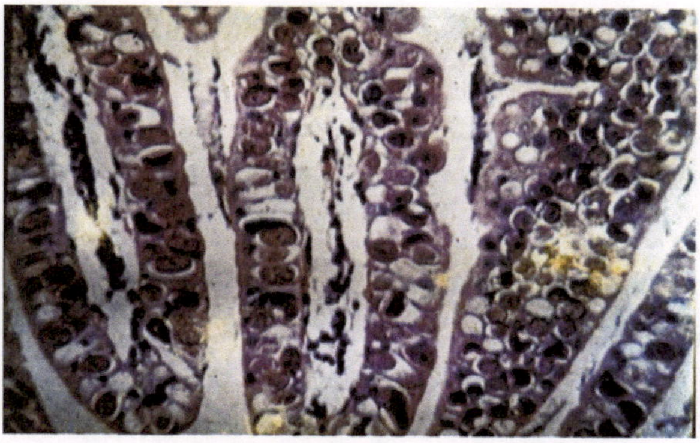

Fig. 9.4: Coccidia in epithelium of intestinal villi of a calf.

Etiology

- Cattle
    - *Eimeria bovis*
    - *E. zuernii*
- Sheep and goats
    - *E. ovina*
    - *E. parva*
    - *E. intricata*
- Pigs
    - *E. scrofae*
    - *E. suis*
    - *E. scabra*
- Equines
    - *E. leuckarti*
    - *Klossiella equi*

Pathogenesis

Oocysts are taken through contaminated water/feed which germinate and liberate the sporozoites. Sporozoites infect the epithelium of intestine and forms schizonts and merozoites that causes damage to intestines leading to haemorrhage. After formation of gametes and fertilization oocysts are again formed and released through stool.

Characteristic Symptoms

- Bloody diarrhoea
- Emaciation

Macroscopic features

- Haemorrhage in intestines
- Anemia
- Hepatic lesions and icterus in rabbits

Microscopic features

- Coccidia in the epithelial cells of villi in mucosa of intestine.
- Eosinophilic inflammation
- Haemorrhagic enteritis

Diagnosis

- Symptoms and lesions
- Demonstration of coccidial parasites in stool, or intestinal tissue sections.

Sarcosporidiosis

Sarcosporidiosis is a protozoan parasitic disease of animals caused by several species of sarcocystis and characterized by presence of cysts in skeletal and cardiac muscles without much inflammatory reaction (Fig. 9.5).

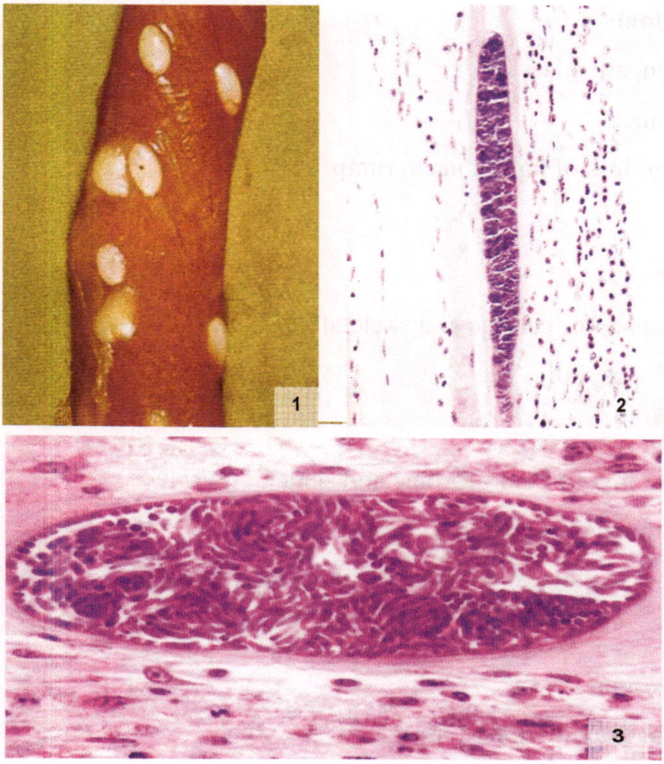

Fig. 9.5: Scarcosporidiosis in animals- (1) Sarcocysts in oesophagus and (2&3) Microscopic features of sarcocysts filled with trophozoites.

Etiology

- *Sarcocystis cruzi*- Cattle
- *S. gigantean*- Sheep
- *S. canis*- Dogs
- *S. capracanis*- Goat

Pathogenesis

On ingestion the sarcocystis enter through blood vessel by damaging the endothelial cells of arteriols and capillaries leading to haemorrhage and anemia, fever occurs during parasitemia and the parasite lodged in muscles.

Characteristic Symptoms

- Fever, emaciation, anemia
- 'Rat tail' appearance
- Muscle twitching, loss of hair in neck, rump
- Abortion

Macroscopic features

- Sarcocyt on oesophagus, cardiac and skeletal muscle
- Loss of hairs on neck, tail

Microscopic features

- Sarcocysts distort myofibrils in cardiac and skeletal muscle
- No or mild inflammatory reaction
- Rupture of sarcocyte may cause granulomatous inflammation

Diagnosis

- Symptoms and lesions
- Histopathological examination of muscles.

Schistosomiasis

Schistosomiasis is a parasitic disease of animals caused by blood fluke characterized by formation of granulomatous pseudo tubercle, cercarial dermatitis and nasal granuloma (Fig. 9.6).

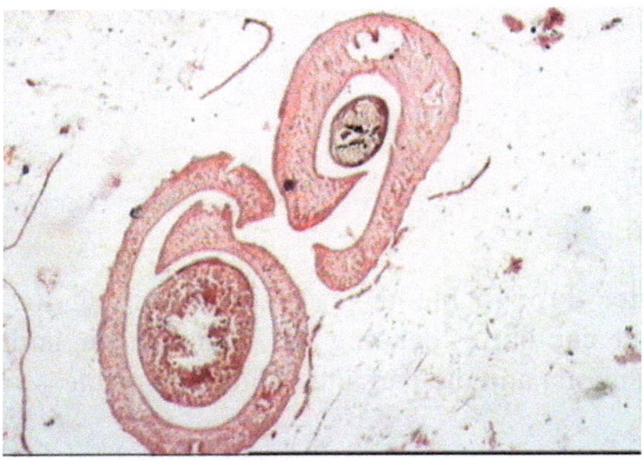

Fig. 9.6: Schistosomes in tissue section.

Etiology

- *Schistosoma nasalis*
- *S. indicum*
- *S. bovis*
- *S. spindale*

Pathogenesis

When the cercariae find a suitable host, they penetrate the skin of susceptible host usually between the hair follicles and converted into metacercariae. Metacercariae enter in small peripheral veins and reach into lungs through venous circulation where they break the lung parenchyma and migrate directly to the liver. In intra hepatic portal system, the flukes grow in size then eventually migrate to the portal, mesenteric or pelvic vein where they attain their adult form.

Characteristic Symptoms

- Dyspnoea
- Epistaxis
- Dermatitis (Swimmers' itch)
- Itching

Macroscopic features

- Granulomatous growth in nasal passage
- Dermatitis
- Haemorrhagic ulcers

Microscopic features

- Micro abscess containing neutrophils and eosinophils surrounding ovum
- Granulomatous reaction-eggs surrounded by mononuclear cells and fibrosis
- Endarteritis, periarteritis

Diagnosis

- Symptoms and lesions
- Examination of lesion and/or blood for flood flukes.

Distomiasis

Distomiasis is a trematode parasitic disease of animals caused by *Fasciola* sp. and characterized by hepatitis, cholecystitis and icterus (Fig.9.7).

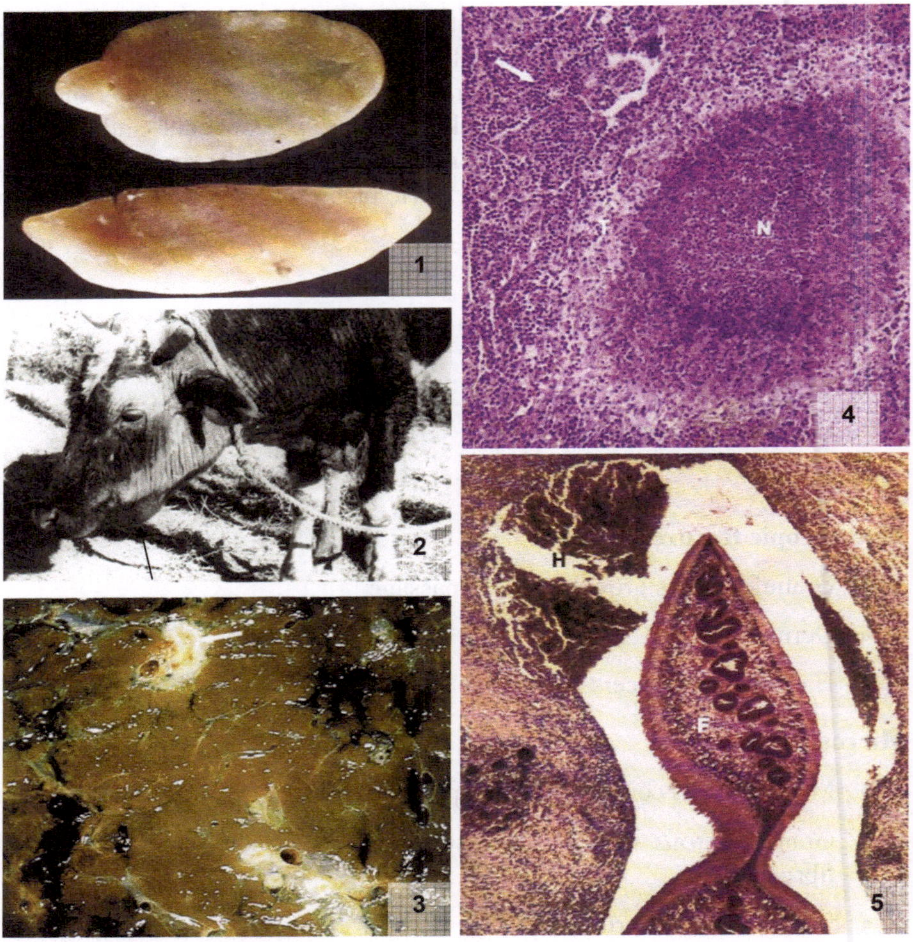

Fig. 9.7: Liver fluke infection in animals- (1) Adult Fasciola sp., (2) Bottle jaw in cattle, (3) Necrotic and prominent bile duct in liver, (4) Microscopic feature of liver central necrosed area(N) surrounded by chronic inflammatory cells and (5) Cross section of parasite in tissue.

Etiology

- *Fasciola hepatica*
- *Fasciola gigantica*

Pathogenesis

The ova of the parasite are disseminated through faeces, which germinate and form miracidium. The miracidium penetrates the body of snails and after several stages, it becomes cercariae which is attached to plants/ vegetation in water source. This form is called as metacercariae, which are ingested by the animals, and reaches in intestine. They penetrate the intestine and migrate to liver to eventually develop in bile ducts and gall bladder.

Characteristic Symptoms

- Anemia, emaciation
- Icterus, diarrhoea/constipation
- Oedema in lower parts of body

Macroscopic features

- Necrotic channels in liver
- Abscess formation
- Presence of parasites in bile duct/gall bladder

Microscopic features

- Infiltration of eosinophils, lymphocytes and mononuclear macrophages
- Fibrosis/cirrhosis of liver

Diagnosis

- Symptoms and lesions
- Faecal examination
- Liver/gall bladder examination during necropsy for the presence of adult flukes
- Demonstration of parasitic antigens in faeces, milk and/or serum using ELISA

Cryptosporidiosis

Cryptosporidiosis is a protozoan parasitic disease of animals characterized by chronic diarrhoea in calves, villous atrophy and infiltration of lymphocytes in mucosa of intestine.

Etiology

- *Cryptosporidium bovis*
- Protozoan parasite just like coccidia

Pathogenesis

Oocysts of cryptosporidia enter in body through faecal- oral route and establish in mucosa of intestine. The merozoites penetrate villous epithelium causing chronic diarrhoea.

Characteristic Symptoms

- Inapparent signs
- Chronic diarrhoea

Macroscopic features

- Congestion of intestines
- Enlargement of mesenteric lymph nodes

Microscopic features

- Villous atrophy
- Infiltration of lymphocyte, plasma cells
- Intra cellular parasite- basophilic
- Necrosis

Diagnosis

- Symptoms and lesions
- Microscopic examination of faecal samples and intestinal scrapings
- Demonstration of parasites in intestinal tissue sections

Ascariasis

Ascariasis is a parasitic disease of animals caused by Ascarid worms and characterized by diarrhoea, jaundice, and obstruction of bile duct, peritonitis and obstruction of intestinal lumen.

Etiology

- *Ascaris lumbricoides*- Pig
- *Toxocara canis*- Dog
- *T. cati*- Cats, dog
- *Neoascaris vitulorum*- Cattle
- *Parascaris equorum*- Horse

Pathogenesis

The eggs or larvae are ingested through feed/water. Larvae invade the intestine and pass through liver to the lungs, enter in bronchi and trachea and then are swallowed to develop adult parasite in intestinal lumen. In cattle larvae may also reach to the foetus through prenatal or trans mammary passage.

Characteristic Symptoms

- Diarrhoea
- Fever
- Constipation
- Jaundice

Macroscopic features

- Presence of adult worms in intestinal lumen
- Hepatitis with sub-capsular fibrosis
- Granulomatous nodules in kidneys, liver, lung, myocardium and lymph nodes
- Larvae may migrate in abnormal host - ***visceral larva migrans*** in man

Microscopic features

- Caseaous hepatitis with fibrosis
- Eosinophilic enteritis
- Haemorrhage in intestines and lungs

Diagnosis

- Symptoms and lesions
- Faecal examination for the presence of parasitic ova
- Presence of parasites in intestines during necropsy

Anchylostomiasis

Anchylostomiasis is a parasitic disease of animals characterized by dermatitis creeping eruptions, anemia, diarrhoea and progressive emaciation. This is also known as ***hook worm disease***.

Etiology

- *Anchylostoma caninum*- Dog
- *Bunostomum phlebotomum*- Cattle
- *B. trigonocephalum*- Sheep, goat
- *Globecephalus urosubulatus*- Pig

Pathogenesis

Eggs are released in faeces, which hatch under suitable conditions into larvae that infect the host through skin penetration or ingestion. Larvae migrate to the lungs and finally reaches in intestine through cough swallowing. During migration, they may penetrate placenta and infect foetus or may appear in milk to infect suckling neonates.

Characteristic Symptoms

- Dermatitis
- Itching on skin
- Coughing
- Anemia, melena
- Progressive weakness

Macroscopic features

- Anemia
- Lobular pneumonia
- Haemorrhage in intestines

- Fibrotic nodules in intestines
- Dermatitis
- Placentitis

Microscopic features

- Haemorrhage in intestine
- Blunting and fusion of villi
- Fibrosis in intestine
- Leucocytic infiltration in lungs and intestines

Diagnosis

- Symptoms and lesions
- Faecal examination for the present of ova
- In intestine adult worms are seen during necropsy
- Demonstration of parasite in tissue sections

Trichostrongylosis

Trichostrongylosis is a parasitic disease of animals characterized by melena, emaciation, progressive weakness, anemia and death.

Etiology

- *Hemonchus contortus*- stomach worm
- *H. placei*- stomach worm
- *Ostertagia ostertagi*- brown stomach worm
- *Trichostrongylus axei*- hair like worm
- *T. colubriformis*- hair like worm
- *Cooperia punctata*- stomach worm

Pathogenesis

Larvae are ingested through feed or water, which penetrate the abomasum and attach with mucosa. They take the blood of host and become mature within 18-19 days. Adult worms live free in lumen but suck blood from the wall of abomasum. Some may pierce the mucosa deep to remain in the wall for longer period that leads to formation of small nodules.

Characteristic Symptoms

- Diarrhoea
- Melena
- Anemia

Macroscopic features

- Nodules in gastric wall
- Haemorrhage in gastric mucosa
- Blood mixed intestinal contents
- Anemia
- Oedema in subcutis
- Abomasum may have large number of worms

Microscopic features

- Mucosa of abomasum becomes haemorrhagic and atrophic
- Infiltration of leucocytes specially of eosinophils

Diagnosis

- Symptoms and lesions
- Faecal examination
- Identification of parasites from stomach during necropsy

Oesophagostomiasis

Oesophagostomiasis is a parasitic disease of animals characterized by diarrhoea, anemia, emaciation, cachexia, prostration and death.

Etiology

- *Oesophagostomum radiatum*
- *O. columbianum*
- These are known as ***nodule worms***

Pathogenesis

Eggs pass through faeces and germinate into larvae in soil. Larvae through contaminated feed/water reaches in gut of animal. The larvae penetrate the intestinal mucosa, moult in sub mucosa and return to the lumen for maturation to become adult worm.

Characteristic Symptoms

- Diarrhoea
- Anemia, emaciation, cachexia
- Prostration and death

Macroscopic features

- Catarrhal enteritis
- Haemorrhage in intestines
- Anemia
- Nodules in sub mucosa
- Parasites in intestines

Microscopic features

- Catarrhal, haemorrhagic and eosinophilic enteritis
- Infiltration of lymphocytes, macrophages and giant cells

Diagnosis

- Symptoms and lesions
- Faecal examination
- Demonstration of parasite in intestinal wall/lumen

Cestodiasis

Cestodiasis is a tapeworm parasitic disease of animals characterized by anemia, haemorrhagic enteritis, abdominal pain, emaciation and diarrhoea. This is also known as ***tapeworm disease*** or ***taeniasis*** (Fig. 9.8).

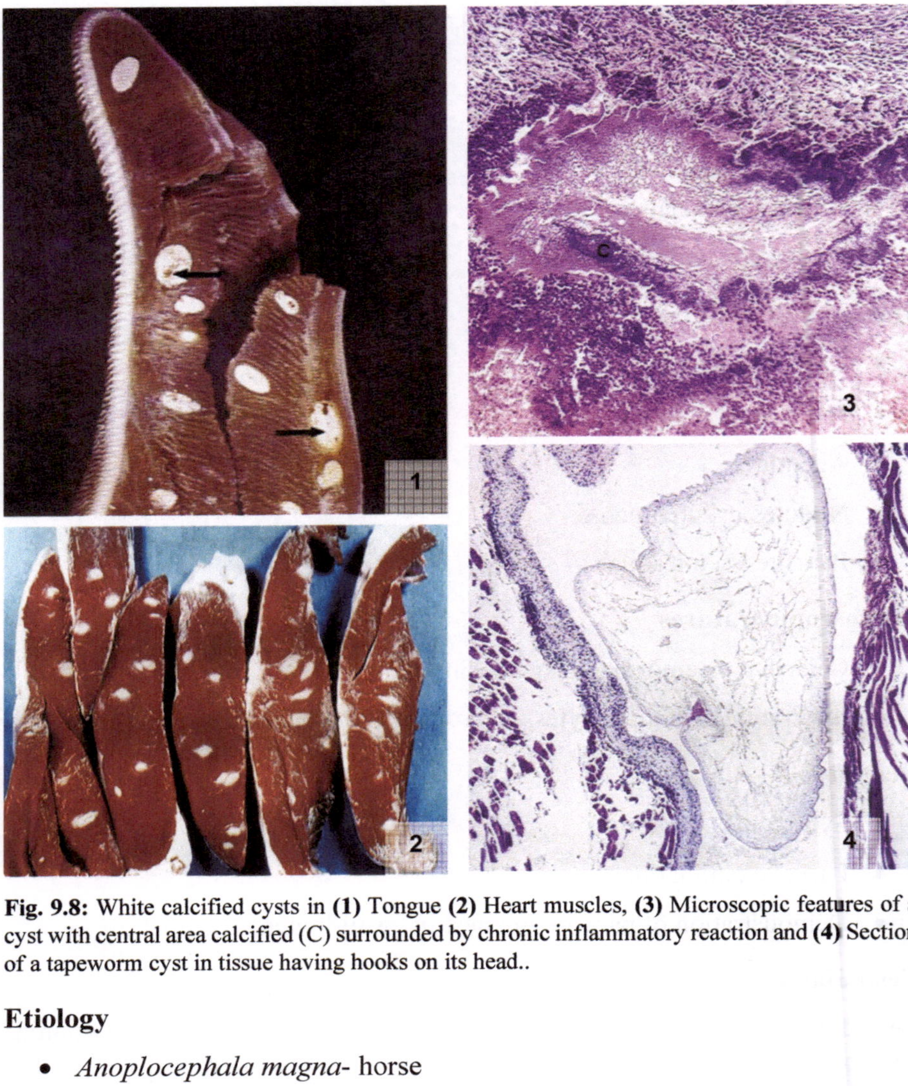

Fig. 9.8: White calcified cysts in **(1)** Tongue **(2)** Heart muscles, **(3)** Microscopic features of a cyst with central area calcified (C) surrounded by chronic inflammatory reaction and **(4)** Section of a tapeworm cyst in tissue having hooks on its head..

Etiology

- *Anoplocephala magna*- horse
- *Moniezia expansa*- sheep, goat, cattle, buffaloes
- *M. benedeni*- sheep, goat, cattle, buffaloes
- *Avitellina centripunctata*- sheep, goat, cattle, buffaloes
- *Diphyllobothrium latum*- pigs, dogs
- *Mesocestoides lineatus*- dogs

- *Dipylidium caninum*- dogs
- *Taenia pisiformis*- dogs

Pathogenesis

Adult tapeworms suck the blood from mucosa of intestines through suckers and hooks causing enteritis and anemia.

Characteristic Symptoms

- Anemia
- Blood mixed faeces, diarrhoea
- Emaciation, progressive weakness
- Jaundice
- Abdominal pain

Macroscopic features

- Haemorrhagic enteritis
- Presence of parasites in intestines
- Blood mixed intestinal contents
- Anemic musculature

Microscopic features

- Hemosiderin in liver and spleen
- Fatty degeneration of brain tissue
- Hemorrhagic enteritis

Diagnosis

- Symptoms and lesions
- Faecal examination
- Presence of parasitic segments in intestine of host

Cysticercosis

Cysticercosis is a parasitic disease of animals characterized by the presence of cysts in different organs of body. This is caused by larval stages of the tapeworms and is also known as ***bladder worm disease***.

Etiology

- *Cysticercus cellulosae* – larvae of *Taenia solium*
- *C. bovis* - larvae of *T. saginata*
- *Coenurus cerebralis* – larvae of *Multiceps multiceps*

Pathogenesis

Cysticercosis is caused by the larval stages of tapeworms, which forms cysts like bladder in different organs including muscles, liver, heart etc.

Characteristic Symptoms

- No characteristic symptoms
- Paralysis of affected organs such as tongue
- Convulsions
- In sheep- this disease is known as *Gid*

Macroscopic features

- Pressure atrophy due to cyst in adjoining tissue/ organ
- Presence of cysts up to several millimeter diameter in muscle, heart, liver, tongue, lungs, brain etc.
- Measly beef or pork

Microscopic features

- Presence of bladder with scolex and hooks in tissue sections surrounded by connective tissue capsules.
- Eosinophilic infiltration

Diagnosis

- Symptoms and lesions
- Presence of cysts in different organs during necropsy

Echinococcosis

Echinococcsis is a parasitic disease of animals characterized by presence of cysts in different organs. This is also known as ***hydated cyst disease***, which is caused by the intermediate stage of tapeworm echinococcus (Fig. 9.9).

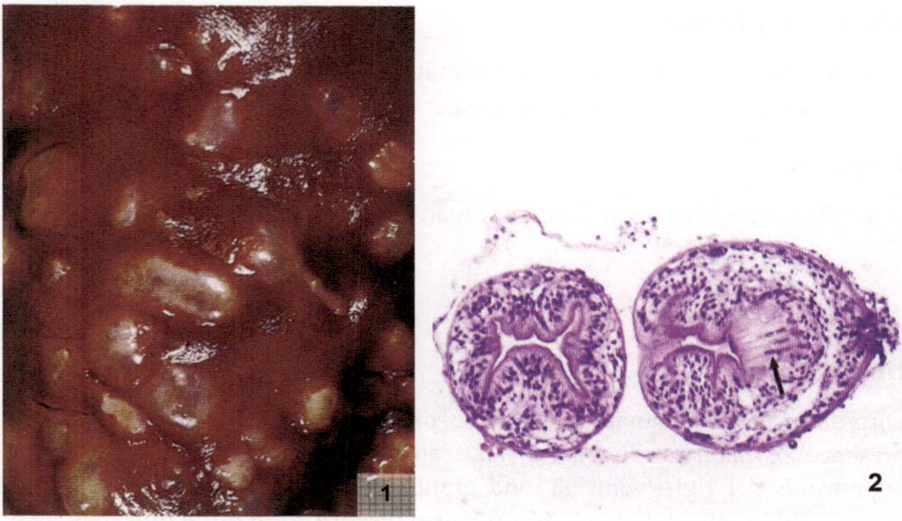

Fig. 9.9: Echinococcosis in animals- **(1)** Cysts in liver, **(2)** Microscopic features of scolices of ecedinococcus in liver section showing hooks (arrow) in one scolex.

Etiology

- *Echinococcus granulosus*
- *E. multilocularis*

Pathogenesis

The cysts may affect organ/tissue which depends on the size of the hydated cyst.

Characteristic Symptoms

- No characteristic symptoms
- Depends on organ involved
- Anaphylactic shock, allergic reaction
- Dyspnoea, diarrhoea, blindness, paralysis

Macroscopic features

- Presence of cysts up to several centimeter in diameter
- Atrophy of adjoining tissue/organ
- Calcified nodules

Microscopic features

- Cysts are surrounded by inflammatory reaction with eosinophils, giant cells and fibrous connective tissue

Diagnosis

- Presence of cysts in different organs/tissue during necropsy
- CFT, DTH, HA test
- Histopathology

Dirofilariasis

Dirofilariasis is a nematode parasitic disease of animals characterized by presence of parasites in blood, heart and arteries causing emboli, ascites, hypertrophy of right ventricle and granulomatous inflammation in visceral organs. This is also kwon as "***Heart worm disease***" or ***canine filariasis***" (Fig. 9.10)

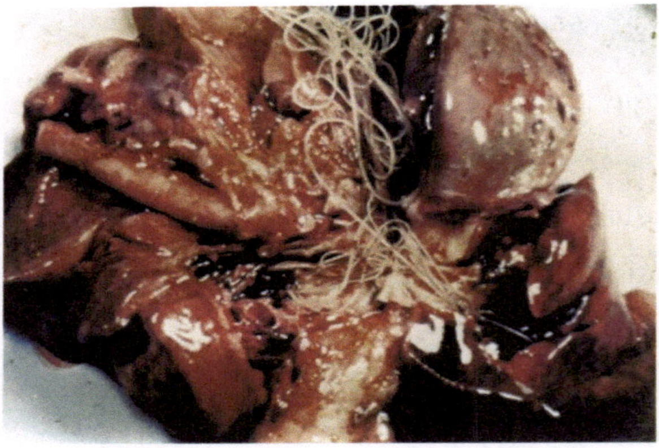

Fig. 9.10: Dirofilariasis in dog- Presence of parasite in heart of a dog.

Etiology

- *Dirofilaria immitis* - dogs
- *D. repens*- dogs
- *Setaria cervi*- cattle
- *S. equina*- Horses
- *Dioctophyma renale*- Pig, dog

Pathogenesis

Transmission of microfilarial worms occurs by biting mosquitoes, in which after some developmental stages, infective larvae enters in body tissues of susceptible hosts. It further develops in muscles, subcutaneous tissue and reaches up to few cm in length and enters in circulation to reach in heart.

Characteristic Symptoms

- Ascites
- Haemoptysis
- Dyspnoea with short breathing
- Weakness

Macroscopic features

- Enlargement of right ventricle
- Presence of worms in heart
- Congestion of lung, liver and spleen
- Ascities
- Pulmonary emboli due to parasite
- Microfilariae in eyes of horse

Microscopic features

- Microfilariae in blood
- Microfilariae in tissue sections with granulomatous inflammatory reaction in kidney
- Cystitis

Diagnosis

- Symptoms and lesions
- Blood examination
- Demonstration of parasite in tissue sections
- Immunodiagnostic tests for detection of parasitic antigen

Dracunculosis

Dracunculosis is a nematode parasitic disease of animals characterized by urticarial rashes, low-grade fever, abscess involving subcutaneous tissue of abdominal wall and legs. It is also known as ***guinea worm disease***.

Etiology

- *Dracunculus medinensis*
- *D. insignis*

Pathogenesis

Infection occurs after ingestion of Cyclops (intermediate host) in water that leads to release of larvae in intestine. They migrate to the connective tissue of abdominal wall, where they become adult and lay eggs, which forms papule and causes itching and oedema.

Characteristic Symptoms

- Intense pruritus, itching in legs and abdominal wall
- Oedema
- Urticaria
- Low grade fever

Macroscopic features

- Oedema
- Papular eruptions on abdominal wall, legs,
- Urticarial swellings
- Subcutaneous nodules

Microscopic features

- Parasites in blood
- Neutrophilic infiltration
- Congestion, oedema in subcutaneous tissue and abdominal wall

Diagnosis

- Symptoms and lesions
- Blood examination
- Demonstration of parasite in tissue sections

Pulmonary Nematodiasis

Pulmonary nematodiasis is a nematode parasitic disease of animals characterized by dyspnoea, coughing, diarrhoea, stunted growth and nodules in lungs. It is also known as ***lungworm disease*** or ***verminous pneumonia*** or ***dictyocauliasis*** (Fig. 9.11).

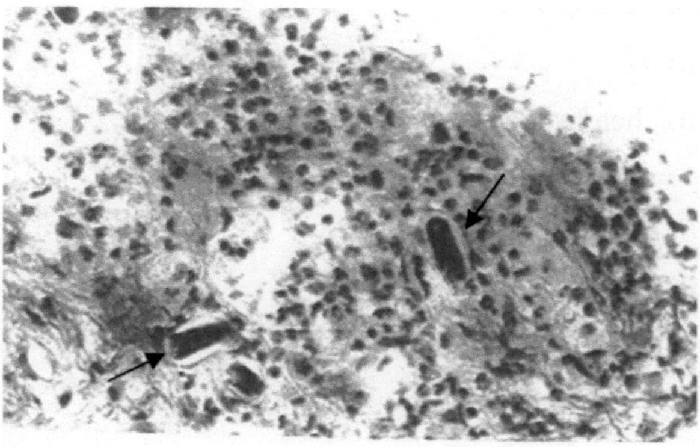

Fig. 9.11: Pulmonary nematodiasis- Presence of worm in lung tissue.

Etiology

- *Dictyocaulus viviparus*- cattle lung worm
- *D. filaria*- cattle lung worm
- *Filaroides osleri*- dog lung worm
- *F. milksi*- dog lung worm
- *Dictyocaulus arnfieldi*- horse lung worm

Pathogenesis

Adult parasites remain in trachea, bronchi and bronchioles and embedded in mucosa. Eggs are laid and swallowed with cough in the gut. The eggs hatch to produce larvae that come with faeces. The third stage larvae are ingested by susceptible animal and penetrate the intestinal wall and migrate to lymph nodes, where they develop 4th stage larvae. By way of lymphatics and pulmonary artery, they enter in bronchioles and bronchi to cause lung lesions.

Characteristic Symptoms

- Hacking cough with dyspnoea
- Diarrhoea
- Retarded growth

Macroscopic features

- Nodules in lungs
- Haemorrhage in bronchiole and alveoli
- Granulomatous pneumonia
- Presence of worms in trachea/bronchiole

Microscopic features

- Presence of parasitic sections in lung tissue
- Eosinophilic infiltration
- Atelectasis and emphysema

Diagnosis

- Symptoms and lesions
- Faecal examination
- Parasite in trachea/bronchiole
- Demonstration of parasitic sections in lung tissue

Equine Strongyloidosis

Equine strongyloidosis is a nematode parasitic disease of equines characterized by verminous arthritis, aneurysm, saddle thrombi, anemia and intestinal infarction (Fig. 9.12).

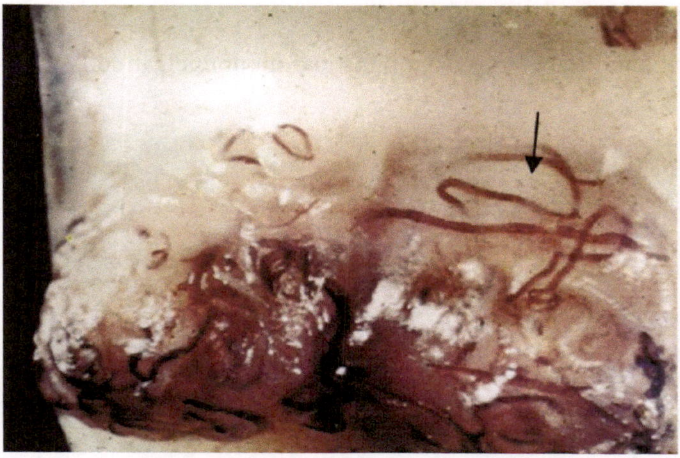

Fig. 9.12: Equine stongyloidosis- Presence of worms in mesenteric blood vessels.

Etiology

- *Strongylus vulgaris*
- *S. equinus*

Pathogenesis

Eggs of parasite pass through faeces; first stage larvae hatched out and develop up to 3rd stage, which are ingested through feed/water. These larvae penetrate intestine, moult in sub mucosa and reach in anterior mesenteric artery. After maturation, the adult parasites return to the intestine particularly in caecum.

Characteristic Symptoms

- Diarrhoea with melena
- Abdominal pain
- Weakness of the legs
- Anemia

Macroscopic features

- Parasites in blood vessel
- Intestinal haemorrhage
- Aneurysm
- Arteritis
- Thrombosis and embolism

Microscopic features

- Parasitic arteritis infiltrated by eosinophils and mononuclear cells
- Infarction
- Proliferation of intima and endothelium
- Haemorrhage

Diagnosis

- Symptoms and lesions
- Demonstration of parasites in blood vessel
- Eggs in faeces- faecal examination
- Histopathological examination

Spirocercosis

Spirocercosis is a nematode parasitic disease of animals characterized by vomiting, oesophageal obstruction and presence of tumour like nodule in aortic wall. This is also known as ***oesophageal worm disease***.

Etiology

- *Spirocerca lupi* in dogs

Pathogenesis

Eggs are released in faeces of infected animal and are taken up by beetles in which they hatch to produce larvae. If eaten by the host, the larvae penetrate the stomach or intestinal wall and following the course of arteries migrating through tunica adventitia and media, the larvae reaches in the wall of aorta and localizes in adventitia of aorta in upper thoracic portion. From here, it can migrate to adjacent oesophagus and penetrate its wall to develop cystic nodule.

Characteristic Symptoms

- Vomiting
- Oesophageal obstruction
- Sudden death

Macroscopic features

- Tumour like nodule in aorta, oesophagus (near cardia)
- Aneurysm in aorta
- Haemorrhage due to aneurysm
- Sometimes nodule in stomach and lungs

Microscopic features

- Worm in tunica adventitia or media of aorta
- Leucocytic infiltration
- Necrotic tract in aorta

Diagnosis

- Symptoms and lesions
- Faecal examination
- Presence of parasite in nodule of oesophagus and aorta

Cerebrospinal Nematodiasis

Cerebrospinal nematodiasis is a nematode parasitic disease of animals characterized by loss of balance, incoordination, paresis of limbs, drooping of ears or eyelid and eosinophilic encephalitis. It is also known as ***neurofilariasis***, ***setariasis*** and ***lumbar paralysis*** and in horses "***Kumri***" (Fig. 9.13).

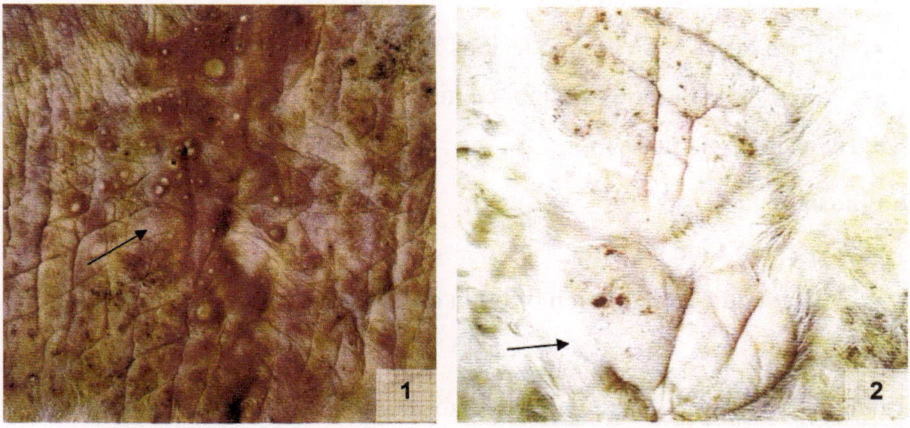

Fig. 9.13: Stephanofilariasis in animals- **(1&2)** Hyperkeratosis, dermatotitis and scab formation on skin.

Etiology

- *Setaria digitata*- sheep, goat, cervids
- *Pneumostrongylus tenuis*- sheep, goat, cervids
- *Micronema deletrix*- horse

Pathogenesis

Adult parasites are harmless while the immature forms occur in brain and spinal cord of sheep, goat and horses.

Characteristic Symptoms

- Paralysis of limbs
- Incoordination of limbs
- Loss of balance

Macroscopic features

- Not well known
- Encephalomyelomalacia
- Presence of parasite in lesion

Microscopic features

- Encephalomyelomalacia
- Eosinophilic infiltration in brain and spinal cord
- Degenerative and necrotic lesions in brain and spinal cord
- Perivascular cuffing of lymphocytes
- Parasite in tissue sections

Diagnosis

- Symptoms and lesions
- Microscopic examination of brain and spinal cord

Trichuriasis

Trichuriasis is a nematode parasitic disease of animals characterized by catarrhal, haemorrhagic or necrotizing typhlitis and colitis. It is also known as ***whipworm disease***.

Etiology

- *Trichuris ovis*- cattle, sheep, goat
- *Trichuris suis*- pig

Pathogenesis

Eggs of parasite are ingested through feed/water, which hatch in intestine and liberate larvae that penetrate the mucosa of caecum and colon.

Characteristic Symptoms

- Diarrhoea with melena
- Weakness and emaciation

Macroscopic features

- Catarrhal / haemorrhagic inflammation of caecum and colon.
- Presence of worms in caecum

Microscopic features

- Catarrhal, haemorrhagic and/or necrotizing typhlitis and colitis
- Parasite in tissue sections
- Eosinophilic infiltration

Diagnosis

- Symptoms and lesions
- Faecal examination
- Histopathological examination of caecum and colon for demonstration of parasitic section

Trichinosis

Trichinosis is a nematode parasitic disease of animals characterized by muscular pain, nausea, vomiting, diarrhoea, fever, oedema of face, urticarial skin eruptions and enteritis. It is also known as ***trichinelliasis***.

Etiology

- *Trichinella spiralis*

Pathogenesis

Uncooked or raw pork products are the source of infection. Infective larvae released from meat and mature in intestine. It enters in intestinal mucosa and through blood stream it reaches in muscles (cardiac, skeletal)

Characteristic Symptoms

- Muscular pain and fever
- Nausea, vomiting and diarrhoea
- Oedema of face
- Urticarial skin eruptions
- Paralysis

Macroscopic features

- Catarrhal enteritis
- Nodule in muscles containing parasite with calcified area
- Parasitic nodules in cardiac muscles

Microscopic features

- Leucocytosis with eosinophilia
- Catarrhal enteritis
- Chalk coloured streaks in skeletal muscles
- Parasite in muscle section

Diagnosis

- Symptoms and lesions
- Parasites or ova in faeces
- Parasitic demonstration in muscles

Stephanofilariasis

Stephanofilariasis is a parasitic disease of animals characterized by dermatitis, hyperkeratosis and scab formation. This is also known as ***hump sore*** or ***ear sore*** (Fig. 9.14).

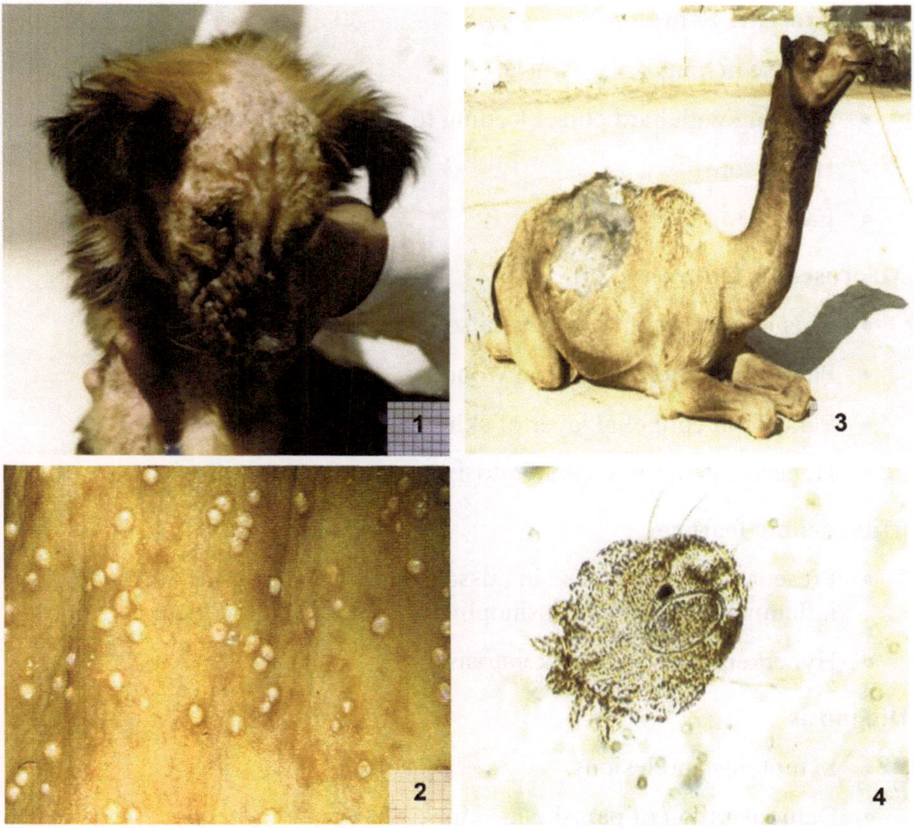

Fig. 9.14: Mange in animals- **(1&2)** Demondectic mange in dogs **(3)** Sarcoptic mange in camel and **(4)** Sarcoptes scabei, cause of mange.

Etiology

- *Stephanofilaria dedosi*
- *S. assamensis*- hump sore
- *S. zaheeri*- ear sore

Pathogenesis

Transmission of parasite occurs through flies. Poor condition of animal and high rainfall are predisposing factors in causation of disease. Disease starts with papular lesions on skin along with itching.

Characteristic Symptoms

- Intense itching
- Rubbing with hard object leading to haemorrhage and abraded wounds
- Hump sore
- Ear sore

Macroscopic features

- This is verminous dermatitis also known as '***Cascado***'
- Papular eruptions, abrasion wounds
- Parasite in epithelial layer of skin
- Hyperkeratosis and parakeratosis

Microscopic features

- Presence of parasites in tissue sections of skin surrounded by inflammatory cells i.e. eosinophils, lymphocytes and giant cells
- Hyperkeratosis and parakeratosis

Diagnosis

- Symptoms and lesions
- Demonstration of parasite in skin

Mange

Mange is a skin disease caused by arthropod parasite mite and characterized by intense pruritus, loss of hairs, hyperkeratosis and thickening of skin (Fig.43.15 and Fig. 9.16).

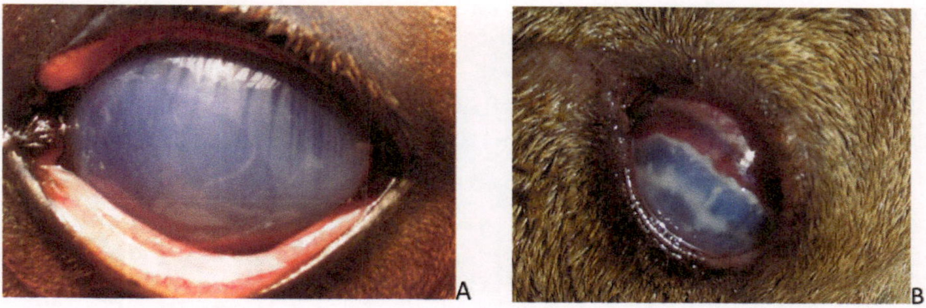

Fig. 9.15: Photograph showing **A.** presence of Setaria spp in conjunctival sac and **B.** corneal opacity in the eye.

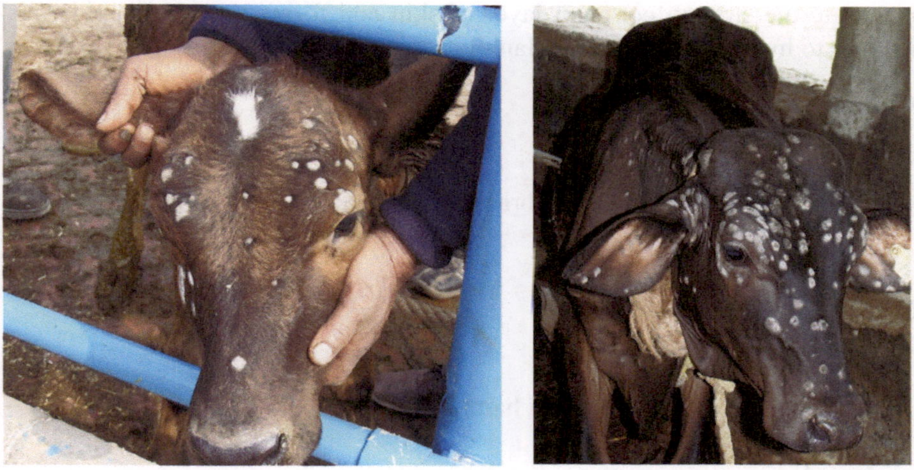

A B

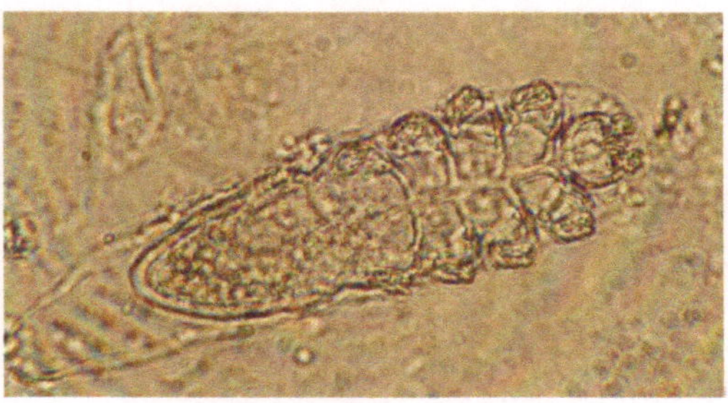

C

Fig. 9.16: Photograph showing- **A & B.** Demmodectic mange in cattle and **C.** Mange mite

Etiology

- Mites- arthropod parasite
    - *Sarcoptes* sp.
    - *Psoroptes* sp.
    - *Demodectes* sp.
    - *Chorioptes* sp.

Pathogenesis

Disease spreads through contact, fomites and rubbing brushes etc. The mites penetrate the stratum corneum layer of skin and forms tunnels in epidermis leading to hyperkeratosis and inflammatory reaction.

Characteristic Symptoms

- Intense itching
- Red papular eruptions or abrasion wounds in skin
- Loss of hairs

Macroscopic features

- Thickening of skin
- Loss of shining of skin and hairs
- Hyperkeratosis
- Scratch wounds

Microscopic features

- Eosinophilic dermatitis
- Presence of mites in skin sections
- Hyperkeratosis and parakeratosis

Diagnosis

- Symptoms and lesions
- Microscopic examination of skin scrapings / tissue

Amphistomiasis

Amphistomiasis is a parasitic disease of animals caused by immature amphistomes and characterized by necrosis of ruminal and intestinal wall, diarrhoea, anemia, dehydration, liver cirrhosis and death. Also known as paramphistomiasis.

Etiology

- Immature helminth – flatworms
- Ruminal flukes – *Paramphistomum cervi*.
- Ingestion of contaminated grass, vegetation.
- Intermediate host - snails.

Pathogenesis

- Metacercariae in grass, ingestion.
- Immature flukes in rumen, attached to the wall of rumen and alimentary tract.
- Causes necrosis, gastroenteritis.

Clinical manifestations

- Diarrhoea, dehydration, anemia.
- Oedema at lower parts of the body.
- Polydipsia.
- Emaciation, death.

Macroscopic features

- Necrosis of ruminal wall, and alimentary tract.
- Presence of immature flukes in rumen.
- Liver fibrosis, Nodular hepatitis.

Microscopic features

- Necrosis of epitheliums is intestines.
- Hemorrhagic entities.
- Necrosis in liver, liver cirrhosis.

Diagnosis

- Symptoms & lesions.
- Presence of amphistome eggs in faecal samples.
- Presence of amphistome in rumen.

Haemonchosis

Haemonchosis is a parasitic disease of animals caused by *Haemonchus contortus* and characterized by diarrhoea, dehydration, oedema in lower parts of body, anemia and death.

Etiology

- *Haemonchus contortus*
- Blood sucking nematode of abomasum.

Pathogenesis

- Ingestion, faecal - oral route of infection.
- Larvae at Pasture – ingestion – attached to the wall of abomasum.
- Suck blood from abomasum leading to anemia, dehydration and oedema at lower parts of body.

Clinical manifestations

- Diarrhoea, melena, oedema at lower parts of body.
- Dehydration, anemia, Pale mucous membranes.
- Sudden death.

Macroscopic features

- Abomasitis.
- Presence of 2 cm long parasite is abomasum.
- Anemia – Pale mucous membrane.

Microscopic features

- Abomasitis, enteritis.
- Decreased total erythrocyte count.

- Presence of parasite in sections of abomasum.
- Eosinophilic in infiltration.

Diagnosis

- Symptoms and lesions
- Faecal examination for parasitic ova.
- Presence of parasites in abomasum during post mortem examination.

10

Pathology of Nutritional and Metabolic Disorders

Equine Rhabdomyolysis

It is also known as Azoturia or Monday Morning Disease. The disease occurs in well fed horse after a spell of inactivity. Suddenly after walking a few steps, the horse is unable to move further and feels pain with intense sweating and hardening of muscles.

Etiology

- Accumulation of lactic acid in muscles.
- High glycogen storage.
- Lack of oxygen supply.

Macroscopic features

- Hardening of muscle just like wood.
- Urine is dark brown with myoglobin – myoglobinuria.
- Tonic spasms in muscles.
- Atrophy of affected muscles in chronic cases.

Microscopic features

- Necrosis of muscle fibres
- Oedema.
- Hyaline degeneration.
- Invasion of sarcolemma by macrophages and lymphocytes.
- Degeneration and necrosis of tubular epithelium in kidneys.

White Muscle Disease

Extensive coagulative necrosis of muscles is observed in calves possibly due to deficiency of vitamin E during 6 months of age (Fig. 10.1).

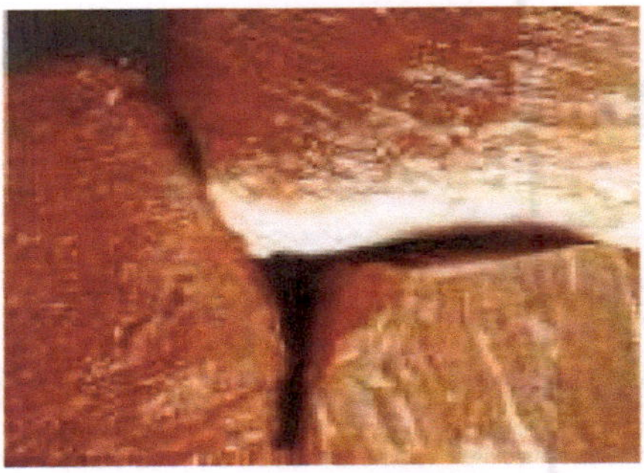

Fig.10.1: Photograph of white muscle disease

Etiology

- Vitamin E deficiency.
- Selenium deficiency.
- Stress.

Macroscopic features

- Colour of muscle becomes pale pink, yellowish red, grey or white (Fig.10.1).
- Muscle becomes dry, inelastic and firm.
- Urine is brown/red or chocolate brown in colour because of myoglobin.

Microscopic features

- Coagulative necrosis of muscles.
- In some muscle cells, cloudy swelling can be observed.
- Neutrophils, macrophages, lymphocytes and eosinophils may be present.
- Calcium may be deposited in necrosed areas.

Fibrous Osteodystrophy

Fibrous osteodystrophy occurs as excessive action of parathyroid hormone on bones and characterized by bone resorption with replacement by fibrous tissue, increased osteoid formation which does not get sufficient minerals for deposition and formation of cysts.

Etiology

- Hyperparathyroidism
- Dietary deficiency of calcium or excess of phosphorus

- Vitamin-D deficiency
- Excessive bran feeding (Disease in horses of flour millers).

Macroscopic features

- Lack of calcification in bone
- Resorption of calcium from bone, fibrosis
- Bone becomes shoft, flexible and deformed
- Rubbery jaw due to involvement of facial bones

Microscopic features

- Fibrous tissue hyperplasia in bones.
- Enlargement of Haversian canals.
- Boney tissue is replaced by fibroblasts, with osteoclastic giant cells lining the remaining bone tissue.

Rickets

Rickets is failure of adequate deposition of calcium in bones of growing animals caused by deficiency of calcium and vitamin D and is characterized by bending of limbs, enlargement of ends of long bones and skeletal deformities (Fig. 10.2).

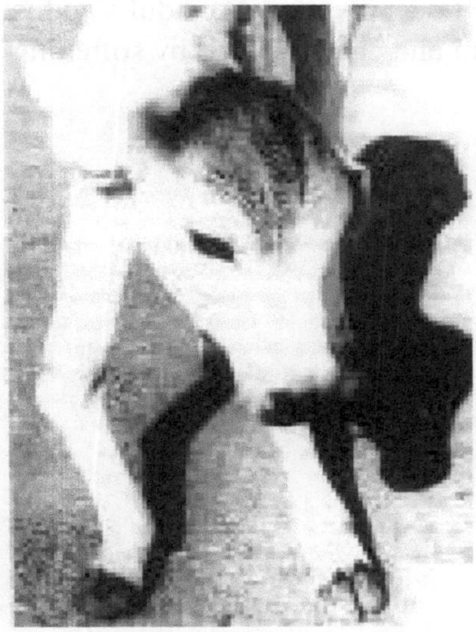

Fig. 10.2: Photograph of calf showing rickets

Etiology

- Vitamin D deficiency.
- Calcium deficiency.
- Deficiency of phosphorus.

Macroscopic features

- Bending of legs, bow legs.
- Pot belly.
- Enlarged costochondral articulation.
- Softening of bones.

Microscopic features

- Increase in proliferating cartilage adjacent to the area of ossification and its disorderly arrangement.
- Disorderly penetration of cartilage by blood vessels.
- Increased area of uncalcified osteoid tissue
- Fibrosis of marrow.

Osteomalacia

Osteomalacia is also known as adult rickets. It occurs in bone of adults and is caused by deficiency of vitamin D and calcium and characterized by softening of bones.

Etiology

- Vitamin D deficiency.
- Calcium-phosphorus ratio disturbance.

Macroscopic features

- Softening of bones.
- Irregular diffuse thickening of bones.
- Bone deformities.

Microscopic features

- Increase in osteoid tissue with failure of calcification.
- Increase in osteoclastic activity.

PICA

Pica is eating of non-food materials like mud, stone, wood etc. by animals due to phosphorus deficiency and characterized by the presence of non-food materials in stomach during post mortem examination (Fig.10.3).

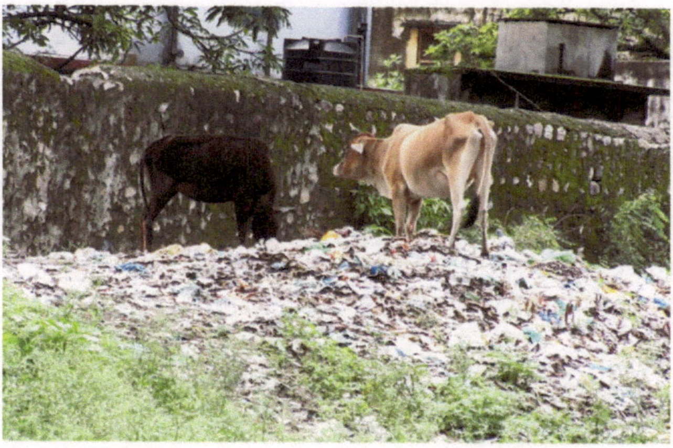

Fig. 10.3: Pica (Eating of non- food materials) in animals

Etiology

- Phosphorus deficiency.
- Rabies – rabid dogs also eat non–food materials.

Pathogenesis

- Though exact cause of pica is not clear, it is thought to be due to phosphorus deficiency and sometimes with heavy parasitic load in the gut.
- Animals eat non - food materials.

Clinical manifestations

- Eating of non - food materials.
- Serum deficient in phosphorus content.
- Faecal examination may reveal heavy parasitic load in gut.

Macroscopic factures

- Dried, weak, emaciated carcass.
- Presence of non - feed material in stomach – stones, mud, wood etc.
- Heavy parasitic load in gut.

Microscopic features

- Parasitic gastroenteritis.
- Eosinophilia.

Diagnosis

- Symptoms & lesions.
- Examination of serum for phosphorus content.

Rheumatism like syndrome

Rheumatism like syndrome is lameness is animals particularly with hind legs possibly due to deficiency of phosphorus.

Etiology

- Phosphorus deficiency.

Pathogenesis

- Due to green revolution, there is imbalance of soil nutrients leading to phosphorus deficient soil in most part of the county.
- Fodder, grains and feed become deficient in phosphorus.
- That leads to deficiency in animals of the area causing lameness in hind legs.

Clinical Mani gestations

- Lameness in hind legs.
- Animals put their legs with jerks.
- Mainly Buffaloes and camels affected.

Macroscopic features

- Not Reported.

Microscopic features

- Not Reported.

Diagnosis

- Symptoms.
- Examination of serum, soil, and fodder for phosphorus content.

Post Parturient Hemoglobinuria

Post parturient hemoglobinuria is a sporadic disease of high yielding cattle caused by phosphorus defeciency and characterized by intravascular hemolysis, hemoglobinuria and anemia.

Etiology

- Phosphorus deficiency.
- Occurs in high yielding cattle just after parturition.

Pathogenesis

- Phosphorus deficiency occurs in soil due of green revolution, resulting in phosphorus deficient fodder.
- Deficiency of phosphorus in animals leads to destruction of erythrocytes.
- Hemoglobin in urine.
- Anemia.

Clinical Manifestations

- Hemoglobin in urine.
- Anemia – Pale mucous membrane.
- Sometimes icterus.
- Serum deficient in phosphorus content.

Macroscopic feature

- Anemic carcass.
- Red / coffee color urine in urinary bladder.

Microscopic feature

- Intravascular homolysis.
- Erythrophagocytosis.
- Bright brown pigment – hemosidrin in spleen.

Diagnosis

- Symptoms.
- Urine analysis – hemoglobinuria.

Milk fever

Milk fever is a non - infectious disease of high yielding cattle caused by hypocalcimia and characterized by restlessness, tremors, ear twiching, ataxia, prostration, paralysis and death. It is also known as post parturient hypocalcaemia, milk sickness etc.

Etiology

- Usually occurs after parturition.
- Deficiency of calcium.

Pathogenesis

- After parturition - increased demand of calcium for milk production.
- Calcium mobilized from bones.
- Animal becomes weak, not able of stand.
- Lying down, Paralysis, Death.

Clinical Mani gestations

- Restlessness, tremors, ataxia, sternal recumbancy.
- Temperature subnormal, cold extremities.
- Paralysis, tachycardia, loss of consciousness.

Macroscopic features

- No Characteristic lesion.
- Food contents may be present at larynx.

- Oedema of trachea and bronchi
- Aspiration pneumonia.

Microscopic features

- No Characteristic lesions.
- Pneumonia, tracheitis, bronchitis.

Diagnosis

- Symptoms.
- Serum examination for calcium – hypocalcimia.

Grass Tetany

Grass tetany is a metabolic disease of cattle and sheep caused by hypomagnesimia and characterized by irritability, in coordination, staggering, coma and death. It is also known as **grass taggers**, **winter tetany** or **hypomagnesimic tetany**.

Etiology

- Magnesium deficiency in grass / forage.
- Hypomagnesimia.

Pathogenesis

- Hypomagnesimia leads to nervous signs, coma and death.

Clinical manifestations

- Hyperirritability, in coordination, staggering.
- Collapse, coma, death.

Macroscopic features

- No characteristics gross lesion.

Microscopic features

- No characteristics microscopic lesion.

Diagnosis

- Symptoms.
- Serum magnesium low levels - hypomagnesimia.

Pregnancy toxaemia

pregnancy toxaemia is a metabolic disorder of sheep coursed by increased energy requirement at late stage of pregnancy and characterized by *hypoglycemia*, hyperketonemia, neurons disorders and death.

Etiology

- Pregnancy with multiple fetuses.
- Increased energy requirement.
- Low glucose availability.

Clinical Manifestation

- Depression, weakness.
- Tremors, Blindness, Ketoacidosis.
- Lying down – lateral recumbancy.
- Death.

Macroscopic features

- Foetal death in uterus.
- Fatty liver.

Microscopic features

- Fatty changes in liver.

Diagnosis

- Symptoms.
- Clinical Pathology.
- Hypoglycemia, Hypocalcaemia.
- Hyperkalemia, hypomagnesaemia.
- Ketone bodies (Beta hydroxyl butyrate in urine).

Acidosis

Acidosis is a metabolic disorder of ruminants, particularly cows caused by excessive carbohydrate in diet and characterized by reduced pH of rumen (pH 5.5), atony and death.

Etiology

- Excessive carbohydrate intake.
- Mostly seen in Gausalas where Gau grass in given in the form of jaggery or wheat flour.

Clinical Manifestations

- Excessive carbohydrate – acute acidosis – death.
- Sub acute acidosis – depression, lethargy, weight loss, death.
- Lameness.

Macroscopic features

- pH of rumen is less than 5.5 (normal 6.5 – 7.0).
- Presence of large quantity of volatile fatty acids and lactic acid.
- Ruminitis.
- Abscess in liver.
- Pneumonia.

Microscopic features

- Ruminitis.
- Suppurative hepatitis
- Pneumonia.

Diagnosis

- History – Symptoms and lesions.
- Rumen PH.

Ketosis (Aetonemia)

Ketosis is a metabolic disorder of cattle, caused by increased energy demand than in take (negative energy balance) and characterized by hypoglycemia, reduced milk production, Ketonemia and ketonuria.

Etiology

- Increased energy requirement then intake.
- Energy deficiency – negative energy balance.

Pathogenesis

- High milk producing animals have high energy requirement.
- Low energy intake leading to development of increased ketone production than utilization.
- Ketonemia, ketonuria.

Clinical Manifestations

- Reduced milk yield, depression, weight loss.
- Ketonemia, ketonuria.
- Lever, nervous signs.

Macroscopic features

- Fatty liver.
- Abdominal displacement.
- Sweet smell from internal organs during P.M. examination.

Microscopic features

- Fatty charges in liver.
- Metritis.
- Ketone bodies in urine, milk.

Diagnosis

- Symptoms.
- Presence of Ketone bodies is blood and urine.
- Ketone bodies: acetoaetate, Beta hydroxy butyrate and acetone.

Sway bock (Enzootic Ataxia)

Sway back occurs in lambs due to feeding of sugar beet top silage to ewes during pregnancy and characterized by nervous signs and encephalopathy.

Etiology

- Copper deficiency.
- Due to feeding of sugar beet top silage to ewes during pregnancy.

Pathogenesis

- Copper deficiency in diet or feeding of sugar beet top silage.
- Interaction of Cu, Mo and S, which makes copper unavailable for absorption.
- Improper synthesis of myelin sheath.
- Nervous tissue damage due to hypocuprosis.
- Myelopathy, neuropathy and encephalopathy.

Clinical Manifestations

- Incoordination.
- Paralysis of hind legs.
- Blindness.
- Prostration.

Macroscopic features

- Vacuolation in brain and spinal cord.
- Encephalomalacia.

Microscopic features

- Chromalolysis.
- Vacuolation in brain neurons.
- Necrosis of brain stem.
- Demyelination of nerve fibres.
- Lack of inflammatory cells.

Diagnosis

- Symptoms and lesions.
- Detection copper levels in tissue / blood.

Pathology of Nutritional Disorders

Malnutrition causes disease in animals either due to deficiency or excess of nutrients. It is very difficult to diagnose the nutritional causes and sometimes it is not possible to find a precise cause as in case of infectious disease because functions of one nutrient can be compensated by another in cell metabolism. Experimental production of nutritional deficiency is not identical to natural disease. When tissue concentration of nutrient falls down to the critical level, it leads to abnormal metabolism and the abnormal metabolites present in tissues can be detected in urine and faeces. First changes of nutritional deficiency are recorded in rapidly metabolizing tissues e.g. skeletal muscle, myocardium and brain. Immature animals are more susceptible to nutritional disease. e.g. calves, chicks, piglets etc.

Types of deficiency

- Acute/chronic e.g. thiamine deficiency in pigs.
- Multiple deficiencies: e.g. poor quality food.
- Nutritional imbalance: e.g. imbalance in calcium: phosphorus (2:1) ratio.
- Protein malnutrition: e.g. malabsorption.
- Calorie deficiency: e.g. Loss of fat/ muscle wasting.

Factors responsible for nutritional deficiency

- Interference with intake e.g. anorexia, G.I. tract disorders.
- Interference with absorption e.g. intestinal hypermotility, Insoluble complexes in food (Fat/Calcium)
- Interference with storage e.g. hepatic disease leads to deficiency of vit. A.
- Increased excretion e.g. polyuria, sweating and lactation
- Increased requirement e.g. fever, hyperthyroidism and pregnancy
- Natural inhibitors e.g. presence of thiaminases in feed, leads to thiamine deficiency.

Calorie deficiency

Calorie deficiency in animals occurs due to food deprivation or starvation.

Food deprivation

Dietary deficiency of food in terms of quantity/quality leads to emaciation, loss of musculature, atrophy of fat, subcutaneous oedema, cardiac muscle degeneration and atrophy of viscera including liver and pancreas. The volume of hepatocytes reduced by 50% and mitochondrial total volume also reduced by 50%.

Starvation

Starvation is the long continued deprivation of food. It is characterized by fatty degeneration of liver, anemia and skin diseases. Young and very old animals are more susceptible to starvation while in pregnant animals it causes retarded growth of foetus. In animals, following changes can be seen due to starvation.

Intestinal involution

Absorptive surface is reduced with shrunken cells and pyknotic nuclei. Villi become shorter and show atrophy.

Atrophy of muscles

There is decrease in muscle mass.

Lipolysis

Increased cortisol leads to increased lipolysis resulting in formation of fatty acids in liver which in turn converts into ketones used by brain.

Gluconeogenesis

In early fasting blood glucose level drops down. The insulin level becomes low while glucagon goes high in starvation. The glucose comes from skeletal muscle, adipose tissue and lymphoid tissue during starvation. Twenty-four hours of food deprivation causes reduction in liver glycogen and blood glucose. Fatty acid from adipose tissue forms glucose and in mitochondria after oxidation it forms acetoacetate, hydroxybutyrate and acetone. These are also known as ketone bodies and are present in blood stream during starvation. This state is also known as ketosis e.g. ketosis/acetonemia in bovines. Lack of glucose in blood leads to oxidation of fatty acids which form ketone bodies as an alternate source of energy. They are normal/ physiological at certain level but may become pathological when their level is high.

Clinically it is characterized by anorexia, depression, coma, sweet smell in urine. Concentration of acetone increases in milk, blood and urine along with hyperlipimia and acidosis. A similar condition also occurs in sheep known as pregnancy toxaemia which is characterized by depression, coma and paralysis. This situation occurs when many foetus are present in uterus. There are fatty changes in liver, kidneys, and heart, with subepicardial petechiae or echymosis.

Protein deficiency

Generally, protein deficiency does not occur. However, the deficiency of essential amino acids has been reported in animals when certain ingredients are deficient in certain amino acids. e.g. maize is deficient in lysine and tryptophan that leads to slow growth; peanuts and soybean are deficient in methioine. Protein deficiency is characterized by hypoproteinemia, anemia, poor growth, delayed healing, decreased or cesation of cell proliferation, failure of collagen formation, atrophy of testicles and ovary, atrophy of thymus and lymphoid tissue.

Deficiency of Lipids

Generally, there is no deficiency of fat in animals. However, essential fatty acids, including linolenic acid, linoleic acid and arachdonic acid, deficiency may occur which causes dermatoses in animals. Fat has high calorie value and it is required in body because there are certain vitamins soluble in fat only.

Deficiency of Water

Deficiency of water may lead to dehydration and slight wrinkling in skin. Deficiency may occur due to fever, vomiting, diarrhoea, haemorrhage and polyuria, which can be corrected through adequate oral water supply or through intravenous fluid therapy.

Deficiency of Vitamins

Vitamin deficiency may occur due to starvation. There are two types of vitamins viz., fat soluble and water soluble. Fat soluble vitamins are vit. A, D, E and K and water soluble are vit B complex and C.

Vitamin A

It is also known as retinol. It is derived from its precursor carotene. It is found in abndance in plants having yellow pigment, animal fat, liver, cod liver oil, shark liver oil. β-carotene is cleaved in gut mucosa into two molecules of retinol (Vit. A aldehyde) which, after absorption, is stored in liver. Bile salts and pancreatic juice are responsible for absorption of vit. A from gut. Deficiency of vit. A occurs due to damage in liver. Vit. A deficiency may lead to following disease conditions:

Squamous metaplasia of epithelial surfaces in esophagus, pancreas, bladder and parotid duct, which is considered pathognomonic in calves. Destruction of epithelium/ goblet cell in respiratory mucosa is generally replaced by keratin synthesizing squamous cells in vit. A deficient animals. There are abnormal teeth in animals due to hypoplasia of enamel and its poor mineralization. Vitamin A deficiency is also associated with still birth and miscarriages in pigs. It causes night blindness (Nyctalopia) in animals. Due to deficiency of Vit. A there are recurrent episodes of conjunctivitis/ keratitis. In poultry, there is distention of mucous glands, which opens in pharynx and esophagus because of metaplasia of duct epithelium leading to enlargement of esophageal glands due to accumulation of its secretions. The glands become spherical, 1-2 mm dia. over mucosa. It is considered pathognomonic for hypovitaminosis A. and is known as Nutritional roup (Fig. 10.4 a&b). Inflammation of upper respiratory tract led to coryza. Urinary tract of cattle, sheep and goat suffers due to formation of calculi, which may cause obstruction in sigmoid flexure of urethra in males. Such calculi are made up of desquamated epithelial cells and salts and the condition is known as urolithiasis. Deficiency of vit. A may also lead to in abnormal growth of cranial bones and there may be failure of foramen ovale to grow leading to constriction of optic nerves which results in blindness in calves, increased CSF pressure, blindness at birth and foetal malformations. In sows, piglets are born without eyes (Anophthalmos) or with smaller eyes- (Microphthalmos).

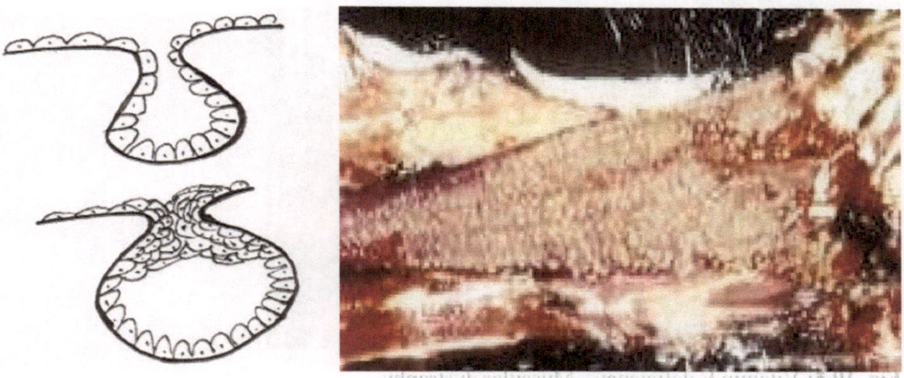

A B

Fig. 10.4: Nutritional roup- vitamin A deficiency

Vitamin D

Vitamin D occurs in three forms viz. vitamin D_2 or calciferol, Vit. D_3 or cholecaliciferol and Vit D_1 or impure mixture of sterols. About 80% Vit. D is synthesized in body skin through UV rays on 7-hydrocholesterol. In diet containing egg, butter, it is found in abundant quantity in milk, plants, grains etc. Active forms of vit. D are 25-hydroxy vit. D and 1, 25 dihydroxy vit D. (Calcitriol) which is 5 to 10 times more potent than former. Vit D is stored in adipose tissue in body. The main functions of vit D are absorption of Ca and P from intestines and kidneys, mineralization of bones, maintenance of blood levels of Ca and P and immune regulation as it activates lymphocytes and macrophages.

- The deficiency of vitamin D is associated with rickets in young animals (Fig. 10.2), osteomalacia in adult animals and hypocalcemic tetany.
- Excess of vitamin D leads to the formation of renal calculi, metastatic calcification and osteoporosis in animals.

Vitamin E (α- tocopherol)

Source of vitamin E is grains, oils, nuts, vegetables, and in body it is stored in adipose tissue, liver and muscles. It has antioxidant activity and prevents oxidative degradation of cell membrane.

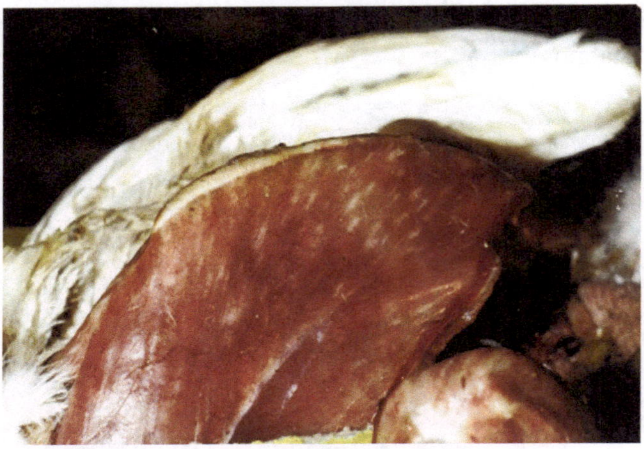

Fig. 10.5: Vitamin E deficiency- Muscular dystrophy

- Deficiency of vit E causes degeneration of neurons in peripheral nerves. There is denervation of muscles leading to muscle dystrophy e.g. White muscle disease in cattle and Stiff lamb disease in sheep and Myoglobinuria in horses. Deficiency of vit. E causes degeneration of pigments in retina and reduces life span of RBC, leading to anemia and sterility in animals. Crazy chick disease (Encephalomalacia) is also caused by vit E deficiency; the chicks become sleepy with twisting of head and neck. There is muscular dystrophy in chickens due to vit. E deficiency (Fig. 10.5).

Vitamin K

Vit. K occurs in two forms namely vit. K_1 or phylloquinone found in green leaf and vegetables and Vit- K_2 or menadione which is produced by gut microflora. Its main function is coagulation of blood. Deficiency of vit K may leads to hypoprothrombinemia and haemorrhages.

Vitamin B

Vitamin B is a water soluble vitamin which has at least 9 sub types including B_1 or thiamine, B_2 or riboflavin, B_6 or pyridoxine, B_{12} or cyanocobalamin, niacin or nicotinic acid, folate or folic acid, choline, biotin and pantothenic acid.

Thiamine

In ruminants, synthesis of thiamine occurs in rumen. Sources of vit. B are pea, beans, pulses, green vegetables, roots, fruits, rice, wheat bran etc. Strong tea, coffee have antithiamine action. It is stored in muscles, liver, heart, kidneys and bones of animals. Thiamine plays active role in carbohydrate metabolism. Deficiency of thiamine may lead to Beriberi disease characterized by Ataxia and neural/lesions. Chastek paralysis in cats, fox and mink and stargazing attitude of chicks due to thiaminase (thiamine deficiency) in meal may be observed. Bracken fern poisoning in cattle and horses may cause deficiency of thiamine due to presence of thiaminase enzyme in bracken fern. Toxicity of thiamine splitting drugs like amprolium, a coccidiostate, may cause polioencephalomalcia in cattle and sheep. Cardiac dialation in pigs has also been observed due to vit. B_1 deficiency.

Riboflavin

Riboflavin is a component of several enzymes and is found in plants, meat, eggs and vegetables.

- Deficiency of riboflavin may cause Curled Toe Paralysis in chicks and swelling of sciatic and brachial nerves (Fig. 10.6).

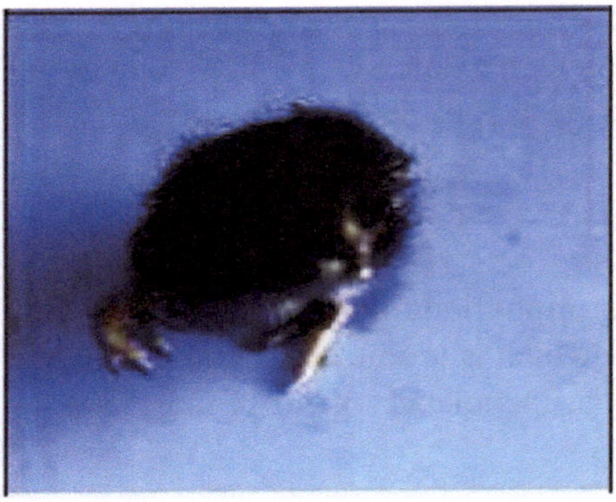

Fig. 10.6: Curled toe paralysis in a chick due to riboflavin deficiency

Niacin

Role of niacin (NAD/NADP, nicotinamide adenine dinucleotide) is in electron transport in mitochondria of cells. It is found in grains, cereals, meat, liver, kidneys, vegetables and plants.

- Deficiency of niacin is associated with skin disorders in man Pellegra; anorexia, diarrhoea, anemia in pigs and mucous hyperplasia, haemorrhage in gastrointestinal tract and black tongue in dogs which is also known as Canine pellegra.

Pyridoxine

It is found in egg, green vegetables, meat, liver etc.

- Deficiency of pyridoxine causes uremia, convulsions, dermatitis and glossitis

Pantothenic acid

- Pantothenic acid deficiency is associated with stunted growth of chicks.

Folate

- Folic acid is required in formation of erythrocytes and hence its deficiency leads to anemia.

Cyanocobalamin

Deficiency of cyanocobalamin may also lead to anemia, as it is also needed in RBC formation.

Biotin

Biotin deficiency causes paralysis of hind legs in calves and perosis in chicks (Fig.10.7).

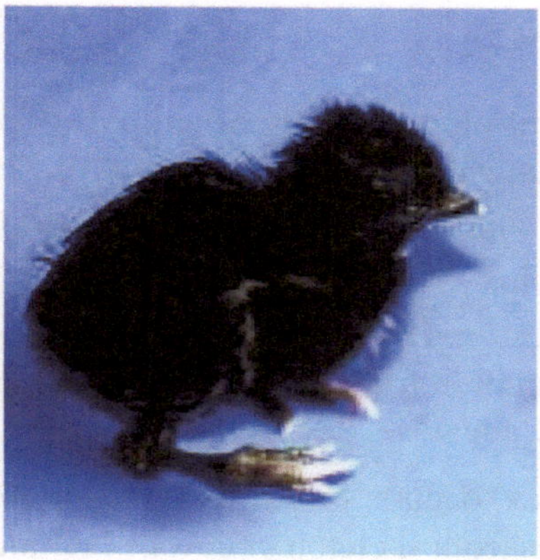

Fig. 10.7: Slipped tendon or perosis in a chick

Choline

Choline deficiency is associated with fatty changes in liver and perosis.

Vitamin C (Ascorbic acid)

It is found in green plants and citrus fruits. Deficiency of vit. C may cause retardation of fibroplasia, scurvy in G. pigs, hemorrhage, swelling, ulcers and delayed wound healing in animals.

Minerals

Various minerals are also necessary for survival of animals. Deficiency of any one of them or in combination may cause serious disease in animals. Some of the important minerals are:

Sodium chloride

Sodium chloride is an essential salt which maintains osmotic pressure in blood, interstitial tissue and the cells because 65% of osmotic pressure is due to sodium chloride. Chloride ions of hydrochloric acid present in stomach also come from sodium chloride.

- The excess of sodium chloride causes gastroenteritis in cattle, gastroenteritis and eosinophilic meningoencephalitis in pigs and ascites in poultry.

- Deficiency of sodium chloride is characterized by anorexia, constipation, loss of weight in sows and pica, weight loss, decreased milk production and polyurea in cattle. Deficiency of salt occurs due to diarrhoea, dehydration and vomiting.

Calcium

Normal range of calcium is 10-11 mg/100 ml blood in body of animals. If it increases above 12 mg/100 ml blood, metastatic calcification occurs, while its level less than 8 mg/100 ml blood may show signs of deficiency characterized by tetany.

Absorption of calcium from gut is facilitated by vit. D. Paratharmone stimulates to raise blood Ca level from bones while calcitonin from thyroid stimulates its deposition in bones and thus reduces blood Ca levels.

- In pregnant cows, calcium deficiency occurs just after parturition. During gestation calcium goes to foetus from skeleton of cows, resulting in weak skeleton of dam. If calcium is not provided in diet, it may cause disease in dam characterized by locomotor disturbances, abnormal curvature of back, distortion of pelvis, tetany, incoordination, muscle spasms, unconsciousness and death. Such symptoms occur in animals when their blood calcium level falls below 6 mg/100 ml of blood and if it is less than 3 mg/100ml blood, death occurs instantly.
- Milk fever is a disease of cattle that occurs due to deficiency of calcium just after parturition. Cow suddenly becomes recumbent and sits on sternum with head bending towards flank and is unable of get up. No gross/ microscopic lesion is reported in this disorder. The calcium therapy recovers the animal immediately.
- The excess of calcium may cause metastatic calcification leading to its deposition in soft tissue of kidney, lungs and stomach.

Magnesium

It acts as activator of many enzymes e.g. alkaline phosphatase. It is required for activation of membrane transport synthesis of protein, fat and nucleic acid and for generation/ transmission of nerve impulses. The normal blood levels are 2 mg/100 ml of blood.

- Dietary deficiency leads to hypomagnesaemia and a level below 0.7 mg/100 ml causes symptoms in calves characterized by nervous hyperirritability, tonic and clonic convulsions, depression, coma and death.

- The post-mortem lesions of magnesium deficiency include hemorrhage in heart, intestines, mesentery and congestion of viscera.
- Microscopic lesions include calcification of intimal layer of heart blood vessels (metastatic) muscles and kidneys. Grass tetany and Grass staggers occurs due to hypomagnesaemia and are characterized by hyper-irritability, abnormal gait, coma and death.

Phosphorus

Normal level of phosphorus is 4-8 mg/100 ml of blood. In bones, it is in the form of calcium phosphate. Deficiency of phosphorus may lead to hypophosphatemia and is characterized by pica, rheumatism and hemoglobinurea.

- Pica is licking/eating of objects other than food. It mainly occurs in cattle, buffaloes and camels, who eat bones, mud and other earthern materials. Such animals have heavy parasitic load in their gut.
- Rheumatism like syndrome is characterized by lameness in hind legs particularly in camels and buffaloes.
- Hemoglobinurea is characterized by the presence of coffee colour urine of animal due to extensive intravascular hemolysis Hemoglobin urea is thus known as postparturient hemoglobin urea.

Selenium

Deficiency of selenium causes hemolysis as it protects cell membrane of RBC and thus its deficiency leads to anemia. Blind Staggers occurs due to excess of selenium.

Iron

Deficiency of iron leads to anemia, which is hypochromic and microcytic but rarely occurs in animals.

Copper

Deficiency of copper results in anemia and steel wool disease in sheep, which is characterized by loss of crimp in wool. Enzootic ataxia with incoordination of posterior limb has been observed in goats.

Cobalt

Vit. B_{12} is synthesized by ruminal bacteria from cobalt in ruminants. Cobalt also stimulates erythropoiesis. Its deficiency may cause wasting disease, cachexia and emaciation in animals. The pathological lesions are comprised of anemia, hemosiderosis in liver, spleen and kidneys.

Manganese

Deficiency of manganese causes slipped tendon in chicken or perosis characterized by shortening of long bones in chickens. It occurs as the epiphyseal cartilage fails to ossify at 12 week of age and epiphysis becomes loose and thus gastrocnemious tendon slips medially. This condition is known as Slipped Tendon or Perosis (Fig. 10.7).

Zinc

Deficiency of zinc may cause parakeratosis in pigs at 10-20 weeks' age. Calcium in diet with phytate or phosphate forms a complex with zinc making it unavailable for absorption leading to its deficiency, which is characterized by rough skin of abdomen, medial surface of thigh, which becomes horny. It also causes fascial eczema in cattle, thymic hypoplasia in calves and immunodeficiency in animals.

Iodine

Deficiency of iodine causes goiter in newborn pigs characterized by absence of hair on their skin. Other signs of iodine deficiencies include abnormal spermatozoa, decreased spermatogenesis, loss of libido, reduced fertility, suboestrus, anoestrus, miscarriages, dystocia and hydrocephalus. Excess of iodine may lead to lacrimation and exfoliation of dandruff like epidermal scales from skin.

Fluorine

Excess of fluorine causes mottling in teeth and bones. The teeth become shorter, broader with opaque areas.

11

Toxicopathology

Cyanide poisoning

Cyanide poisoning occurs in animals due to sorghum and/or other chemicals and characterized by ataxia, incoordination, cystitis, paralysis, and death.

Etiology

- Sorghum – drought resistant varieties.
- Fumigants, fertilizers,
- Pesticides.
- Industrial leakage/waste, electroplating.
- Photographic processes.

Pathogenesis

- Cyanide binds with heme (iron) portion of hemoglobin.
- Arrests the aerobic metabolism.
- Death due to anoxia.

Clinical manifestations

- Ataxia, in coordination, muscular tremors, cystitis, frequent urination, convulsions.
- Paralysis and death.

Macroscopic features

- Cystitis, no blood clot, endocardial hemorrhage.
- Necrosis in central nervous system, ulcers in abomasum.
- Cyanotic mucous membranes of respiratory system.

- Rumen is distended with gas.
- Lungs, liver, spleen and trachea congested.

Microscopic features

- Congestion and hemorrhage in vital organs.
- Cystitis.
- Neuronal degeneration in central nervous system.

Diagnosis

- Symptoms and lesions.
- Cyanide detection in tissues/ruminal contents through chemical tests.

Arsenic Poisoning

Arsenic poisoning occurs in animals due to many different types of arsenic compounds and characterized by diarrhea, colic, shock and death.

Etiology

- Pesticides, ant baits, wood preservatives.
- Malicious poisoning.
- Arsenates for tick control.

Pathogenesis

- Arsenic ingestion, absorption in blood though intestines and bound to red blood cells.
- Distributed to body tissues including liver, Kidneys, heart and lungs.

Clinical Manifestations

- Watery diarrhea tinged with blood.
- Colic.
- Dehydration and death.

Macroscopic features

- Hemorrhagic enteritis.
- Myocardial and endocardial hemorrhage.
- Congestion and hemorrhage in liver, lung, spleen and lymph nodes.

Microscopic features

- Pancytopenia.
- Basophilic stippling.
- Hemorrhage in endocardium, myocardium, liver, spleen, lymph nodes, Kidneys.

Diagnosis

- Symptoms and lesions.
- Chemicals test for detection of arsenic in tissues/blood/ingesta.

Nitrate poisoning

Nitrate poisoning occurs in animals due to feeding of nitrate containing feed like barley, Maize, cauliflower and characterized by dyspnoea, weakness, staggering gait, convulsions, cyanosis and death.

Etiology

- Maize, Sorghum, Barley.
- Cauliflower, Potato, Sugar beet.
- Nitrate containing food materials.

Pathogenesis

- Nitrate broken down into nitrite in rumen.
- Normally it is further broken down into ammonia utilized by rumen microbes in protein synthesis.
- Large quantities of nitrite absorbs in blood binding with heme of rbc causing anoxia.

Clinical Mani gestations

- Dyspnoea, weakness.
- Staggering gait.
- Convulsions, cyanosis, death.

Macroscopic features

- Endocardial hemorrhages.
- Cyanosis, chocolate colour blood.
- Haemorrhagic enteritis.

Microscopic features

- Hemorrhages in internal organs.
- Oedema, hemorrhage in muscles, tongue.

Diagnosis

- Symptoms and lesions.
- Chemical test for detection of nitrate/nitrite in tissues/blood/ingesta.

Lantana Poisoning

Lantana poisoning occurs in animals due to feeding of *Lantana camara* plant and characterized by Sore month, photosensitization, hepatopathy, icterus and death (Fig.11.1).

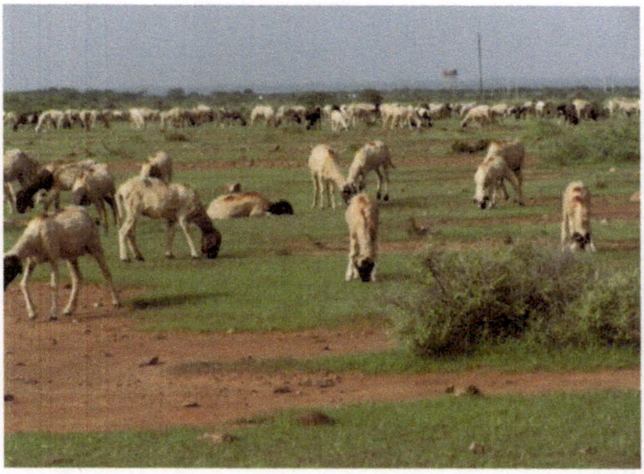

A

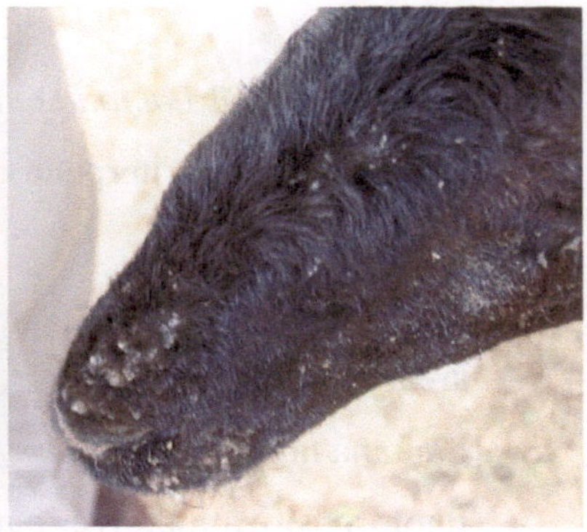

B

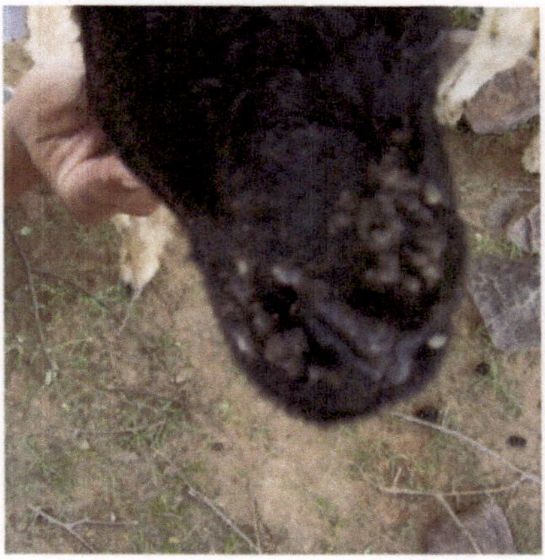

C

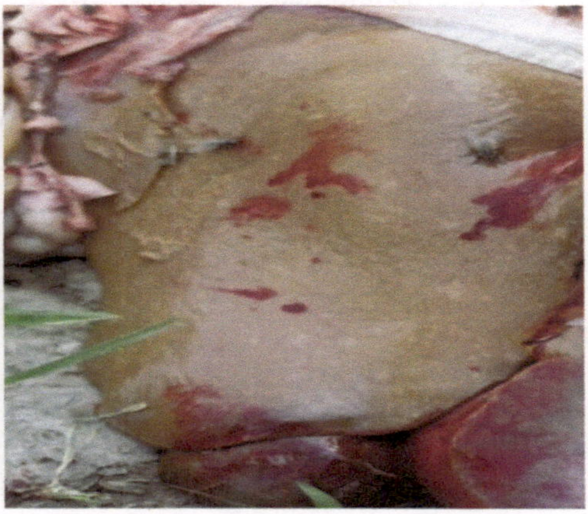

D

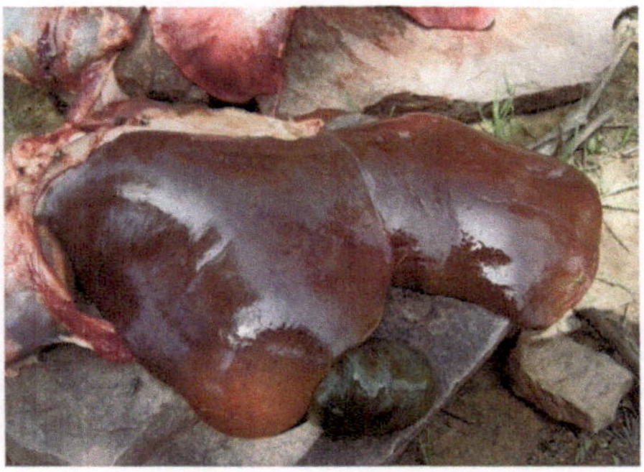

E

Fig.11.1: Lantana poisoning in sheep: A. Sheep grazing in field with new growth of lantana plants just after first rain, B.&C. Presence of scabs on mouth and face, D &E. Icteric liver.

Etiology

- Common weed *Lantana camera.*
- Lantana toxins-Triterpenes acids, lantadene A&B.

Pathogenesis

- Lantana feeding as contaminant of grass or grazing in recently rained areas.
- Lantana taxing in blood.
- Photosensitization, liver damage.
- icterus and death.

Clinical Manifestations

- Sore month – oral ulcers, scabs, allergies at snout, nostrils and mouth.
- Icterus.
- Photosensitization.
- Death.

Macroscopic features

- Yellowish carcass.
- Ulcerative month lesions.
- Neurosis in liver, distended gall bladder.
- Nephritis.
- Undigested plant material in rumen.

Microscopic features

- Skin ulcers.
- Necrosis in liver.
- Hemorrhagic spleen, lymph nodes, muscle.

Diagnosis

- Symptoms and lesions.
- Chemical test for detection of lantana toxins in tissues, blood and ingesta.

Ratti Poisoning

Ratti Poisoning may occur in animals mostly as a malicious poisoning and characterized by sudden death, convulsions, liver failure and vomiting.

Etiology

- *Abrus precatorius* – Ratti – seeds.
- Abrin is highly toxic (0.00015% of body wt – toxic).
- Seed used in human ornaments, measurement of weight.

Pathogenesis

- Introduced in animals by hide seekers through a pin.
- Abrin on introduction in animal body enters in cell and prevents protein synthesis.
- Can inactivate 1500 ribosomes per sec.
- Causes nausea, vomiting, sudden death.

Clinical manifestations

- Hypersalivation, nasal discharge.
- Melena, diarrhoea.
- Vomiting, convulsions, paralysis and death.

Macroscopic features

- No characteristic gross lesion due to sudden death.
- Necrotic liver
- Presence of needle in soft parts of skin/body.

Microscopic features

- Necrosis is liver.
- No characteristic microscopic lesion.

Diagnosis

- Symptoms and lesions.
- Presence of needle in soft parts of body such as vulva.

Strychnine poisoning

Strychnine poisoning occurs is animals as a malicious poisoning caused by baits of strychnine and characterized by nervous signs, convulsions and death within few hours (Fig.11.2).

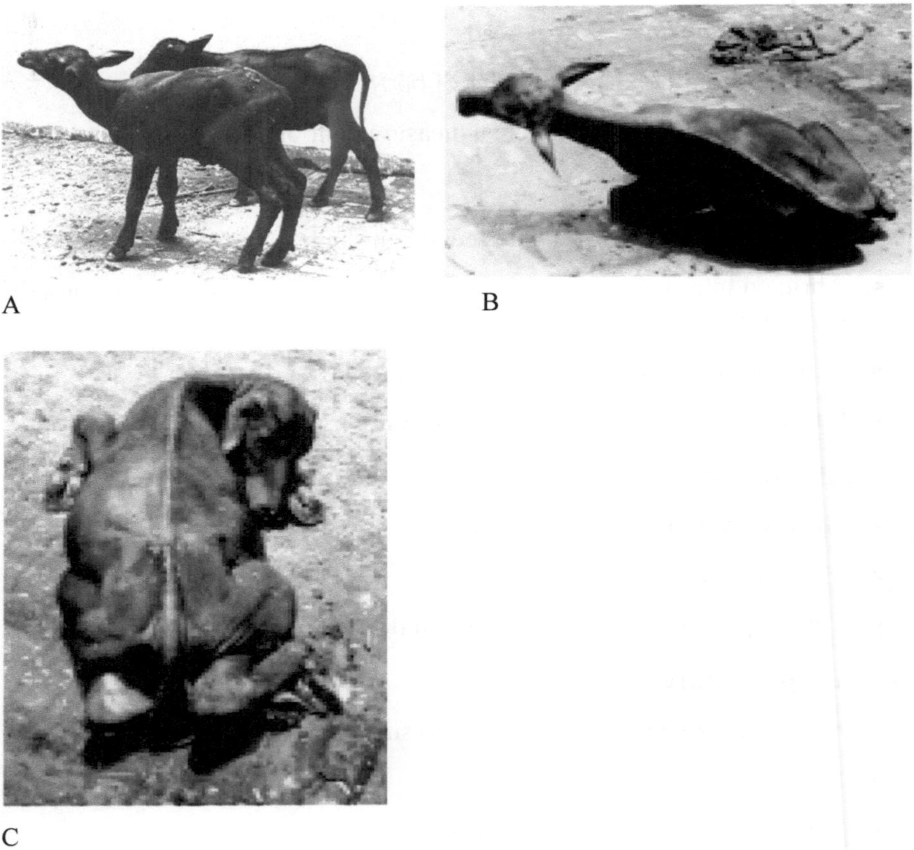

Fig. 11.2: Strychnine poisoning in animals: **A.** Stiffness in legs and neck, **B.** Prostration and staggers and **C.** Torticollis in buffalo calves.

Etiology

- *Strychnos nuxvomica.*
- Strychnine baits are used to kill rodents, dogs and is used as pesticide.
- Malicious use of strychnine baits cause poisoning in animals.

Pathogenesis

- On oral administration, it readily absorbed from the intestines.
- Inhibits neurotransmitter.
- Rigidity is muscles, tonic and clonic spasms.
- Death.

Clinical Manifestations

- Convulsions.
- Tonic/clonic spasms.
- Torticollis.
- Death occurs within 1-2 hr.

Macroscopic features

- Rigor mortis early and rapid.
- Torticollis.
- Endocardial hemorrhage.

Microscopic features

- Hemorrhage in heart, lungs, liver.

Diagnosis

- Symptoms and lesions.
- Chemical tests for detection of strychnine in blood, tissues, ingesta.

Bracken fern poisoning

Bracken fern poisoning occurs is animals due to ingestion of fern along with grazing or fodder and characterized by hematuria, neoplasm in urinary bladder and death (Fig.11.3).

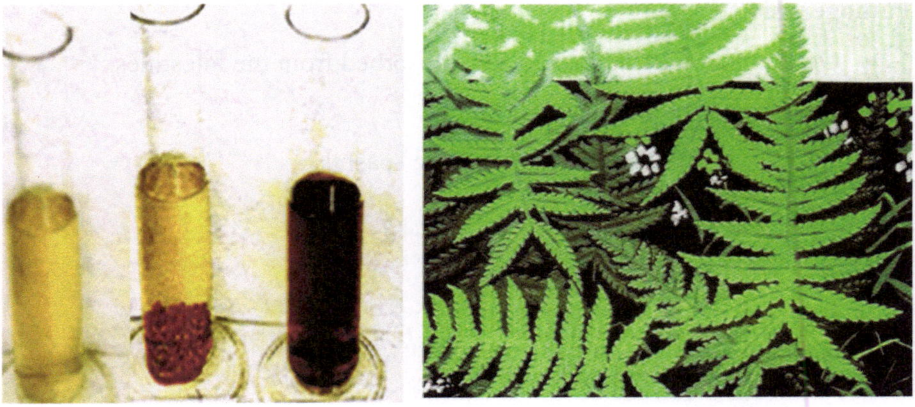

A **B**

Fig.11.3: Bracken fern poisoning in animals: A. Hematuria and B. Bracken fern

Etiology

- Bracken fern – *Pteridium aquilinum.*
- Ptaquiloside – active toxin.

Pathogenesis

- Prolonged ingestion leads to thiamine deficiency and aplastic anemia.
- Hematuria, melena.

Clinical Manifestations

- Blood in urine.
- Bloody diarrhoea.
- Fever, weakening, collapse, and death.

Macroscopic features

- Anemic mucous membranes.
- Tumours in urinary bladder.
- Blood mixed urine – hematuria.

Microscopic features

- Hemorrhage in liver, kidneys.
- Neoplasia in urinary bladder.
- Aplastic anemia.

Diagnosis

- Symptoms and lesions.
- Braken fern identification.
- Detection of Ptaquiloside.

Gossypol poisoning

Gossypol poisoning occurs in animals due to prolonged intake of cotton seed or cottonseed products having excess free gossypol and characterized by hepatotoxicity, oedema in brisket region, gastroenteritis, hemoglobinuria and death.

Etiology

- Cotton Seed (*Gossypium* spp)- Gossypol.
- Prolonged consumption.

Pathogenesis

- Feeding of cottonseed seed or cotton seed products.
- Gossypol in intestines readily absorption reaches to blood circulation.
- Inhibits several enzymatic processes and cause toxicity.

Clinical manifestation

- Hemoglobinuria.
- Diarrhoea.
- Oedema in brisket region, dyspnoea.

Macroscopic features

- Cardiomyopathy.
- Hepatopathy.
- Hemoglobinuria.

Microscopic features

- Necrosis, hemorrhage in liver, kidneys, heart, muscles.
- Hemorrhagic enteritis.

Diagnosis

- Symptoms and lesions.
- Detection of gossypol in blood/tissues/ingesta.

Copper toxicity

Copper poisoning may occur in animals particularly in sheep and is characterized by liver damage, gastroenteritis, anemia, icterus and death.

Etiology

- Copper salts – anti helmintics, mineral mixutre, improper formulation of feed.
- Ingestion of *Trifolium subterraneum* plants.

Pathogenesis

- Copper intake leads to its increased concentration in blood.
- Intravascular hemolysis.
- Hepatopathy, icterus, anemia and death.

Clinical Manifestations

- Diarrhoea, melena.
- Hemoglobinuria.
- Anemia, icterus.

Macroscopic features

- Hepatopathy.
- Gastroenteritis – ulcers is abomasum.
- Icterus.
- Enlarged spleen.

Microscopic features

- Centrilobular hepatic necrosis.
- Necrosis of tubular epithelium in Kidneys.
- In Chronic cases – cirrhosis of liver.

Diagnosis

- Symptoms and lesions.
- Detections of copper in blood and tissues.

Lead toxicity

Lead toxicity occurs in animals due to its excess in environment and is characterized by gastroenteritis, muscle tremors, immunosuppression and death.

Etiology

- Lead based paints.
- Battery disposal.
- Vegetation along road side due to automobile smoke, generator smoke etc.

Pathogenesis

- Lead in blood – Sulfhydryl ion containing enzymes and erythrocytes.
- Capillary damage.
- Immunosuppressive, teratogenic, nephrotoxic.

Clinical Manifestations

- Gastroenteritis – diarrhoea.
- Tremors, convulsions, in coordination.
- Blindness.

Macroscopic features

- Gastroenteritis – presence of paint in gastro intestinal tract.
- Endocardial hemorrhage.
- Enlarged and swollen Kidneys, liver.

Microscopic features

- Basophilic stippling in RBC's in dogs.
- Tubular necrosis in kidneys.
- Intra nuclear inclusions in kidney epithelium.

- Necrosis in liver.
- Necrosis and oedema of white matter.

Diagnosis

- Symptoms and lesions.
- Detection of lead in blood and tissues.

Mercury toxicity

Mercury poisoning occurs is animals as an environmental contaminants of food chain and characterized by gastroenteritis, nephropathy, neuropathy and immunosuppression.

Etiology

- Fish – Bioaccumulation of industrial waste.
- Fossil fuel, thermometers, light bulbs.
- Ayurvedic medicines.

Pathogenesis

- Mercury in gastrointestinal tract causes ulcers.
- In blood – interferes the metabolic activity resulting in nephropathy, neuropathy and Immunopathology.

Clinical Manifestations

- Diarrhoea, Dyspnoea, melena.
- Hematuria.
- Ataxia, in coordination, blindness, paralysis.

Macroscopic features

- Ulcers in gastrointestinal tract.
- Nephropathy.
- Encephalomalacia.

Microscopic features

- Interstitial nephritis.
- Neuronal degeneration and perivascular cuffing in brain.

- Ulcerative gastroenteritis.
- Depletion of lymphoid tissue in spleen.

Diagnosis

- Symptoms and lesions.
- Detection of mercury is tissues/blood/ingesta.

Cadmium toxicity

Cadmium poisoning occurs is animals as an environmental contaminant of food chain and Characterized by nephropathy, pneumonia, osteomalacia, immunosuppression and arthritis.

Etiology

- Cadmium – heave metal contamination occurs in environment due to fertilizers, electroplating, paints, batteries, construction industrial waste.
- Contaminated fodder, water, feed.

Pathogenesis

- Cadmium – respiratory damage tracheobronchitis.
- Blood – Kidneys – renal failure.
- Immunosuppression through damage is lymphoid System.

Clinical Manifestations

- Nasal discharge, rhinitis, bronchitis.
- Gout, Joint Pain.
- Renal failure – oliguria.

Macroscopic features

- Pneumonia, tracheobronchitis.
- Swollen Kidneys
- Osteomalacia.

Microscopic features

- Pneumonia, trachea is, bronchitis.
- Osteoporosis, osteomalacia.

- Nephrosis.
- Depletion of lymphocil cells in spleen and lymph nodes.

Diagnosis

- Symptoms and lesions.
- Detection of cadmium in feed, fodder, water, ingesta, blood and/ or tissues.

Fluoride toxicity

Fluoride poisoning occurs is animals as an environmental pollutant from industrial waste and/or smelting processes and is characterized by sclerosis, exostosis and osteoporosis.

Etiology

- Environmental pollution from industrial waste and /or smelting processes.
- Pesticides – acaricides, rodenticides.
- Fertilizers, mineral supplements.

Pathogenesis

- Fluoride in body causes impaired mineralization of bones and teeth.
- Bone becomes brittle and frazile.
- Dental abnormalities.

Clinical Manifestations

- Tachycardia, dypnoea, clonic convulsions.
- Dental abnormalities.
- Bores more prone to fracture.
- Anemia, hypothyroidism.

Macroscopic features

- Necrosis in liver, Kidneys, lungs.
- Skeletal and dental abnormalities.
- Exostosis.
- Sclerosis and osteoporosis.

Microscopic features

- Necrosis in liver, kidneys and lugs.
- Gastroenteritis.
- Increase in osteoblast activity leading to exostosis.

Diagnosis

- Symptoms and lesions.
- Detection of fluoride in water/fodder/ blood/tissue/bones etc.

Selenium Toxicity

Selenium toxicity may occur in animals due to grazing of selenium containing plants and is characterized by weak hairs, hooves, myopathy and hepatopathy.

Etiology

- Selenium accumulating plants such as Astragalas, Stanleya, oonopsis.
- Mineral mixture high in selenium content.
- Error in feed formulation may also lead to selenium toxicity.

Pathogenesis

- Selenium toxicity also known as blind staggers.
- Watery diarrhea, fever, pneumonic changes.
- Weak hair and hooves.

Clinical Manifestations

- Fever, watery diarrhea, Pneumonia.
- Blind staggers.
- Poor hairs, weak hooves.
- Abdominal pain.

Macroscopic features

- Myopathy, hepatopathy.
- Weak hair, hooves.
- Blindness.

Microscopic features

- Necrosis is liver.
- Pulmonary oedema.
- Extensive hemorrhage in vital organs including kidneys.

Diagnosis

- Symptoms and lesions.
- Detection of selenium in feed/fodder/tissue/blood.

Oxalates Poisoning

Oxalate poisoning may occur is animals due to feeding of oxalate containing plants/ feed and is characterized by weakness, hematuria, tremors, polydipsia and polyuria.

Etiology

- Fruits/vegetable high in oxalate – Spinach, brocoli.
- Posture grass – *Setaria sphacelata.*

Pathogenesis

- Oxalates absorbed from intestine in blood stream causes systemic disorders.
- Insoluble oxalates cause surface irritation on skin and mucous membrane of gastrointestinal tract.

Clinical Manifestations

- Hypersalivation, polydipsia, polyuria.
- Vomiting, diarrhoea, weakness.
- Tremors,
- Hematuria.

Macroscopic features

- Nephrosis, stones in kidneys.
- Oedema, petechiae in sub cutis.
- Anasarca.
- Enlarged lymph nodes.

Microscopic features

- Degeneration and necrosis in Kidneys.
- Oxalate crystals in Kidneys.
- Gastroenteritis.

Diagnosis

- Symptoms and lesions.
- Detection of oxalates in urine, Kidneys.

Pesticide Poisoning

Pesticide poisoning occurs is animals due to malicious or accidental and chronic as environmental pollutant in food chain and characterized by acute death with extensive hemorrhage in vital organs while chronic pesticide poisoning leads to immune suppression and / or autoimmune reactions (Fig.11.4).

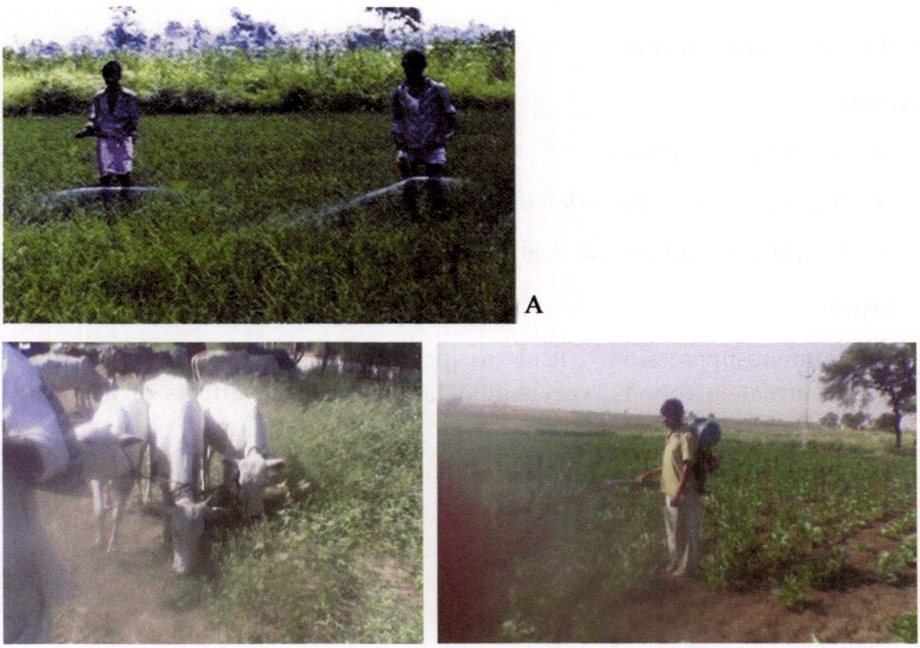

A

B C

Fig.11.4: Pesticide toxicity in animals: A. Pesticide spray on fodder crop, B. Pesticide spray in front of grazing animals and C. Grazing animals in pesticide spray area directly consuming the pesticide.

Etiology

- Pesticides – Insecticide, herbicide, rodenticides, weedicides.
- Mainly of 4 groups: organochlorine, organophosphates, carbamates and Synthetic pyrethroids.
- Spray on fodder crops, washing of equipment / container in water bodies, malicious, accidental.
- Chronic – Bioaccumulation in food chain-fodder, grains, feed, water, air etc.

Pathogenesis

- Acute – malicious/accidental cause nervous disorders and death.
- Chronic in feed chain, enters in body and cause lymphocytolysis leading to immunosuppression.
- Binds with certain body proteins cause autoimmune reactions.

Clinical manifestations

Acute

- Vomiting, Diarrhoea.
- Muscle tremors, constricted pupil, tachycardia.
- Respiratory failure and death.

Chronic

- Immunosuppression – leads to increased susceptibility to infections, recurrent infections, vaccination failure, reduced effects of antibiotic drugs.
- Autoimmune reaction leads to Kidney failure, rheumatoid arthritis, hyperirritability.

Macroscopic features

Acute

- Extensive hemorrhage in vital organs.
- Gastroenteritis,

Chronic

- Atrophy of lymphoid organs.
- Suppressed bone marrow.

Microscopic features

- Lymphocytolysis.
- Depletion of lymphoid tissue in spleen, thymus, bone marrow, lymph nodes.

Diagnosis

- Symptoms & lesions
- Detection of Pesticide in feed/Blood/tissues/ingesta.

12

Pathology of Laboratory Animal Diseases

Tyzzer's disease

Tyzzer's disease is an acute infectious disease of laboratory animals including rats caused by *Clostridium* spp and Characterized by watery diarrhoea, necrotic hepatitis and death (Fig.12.1).

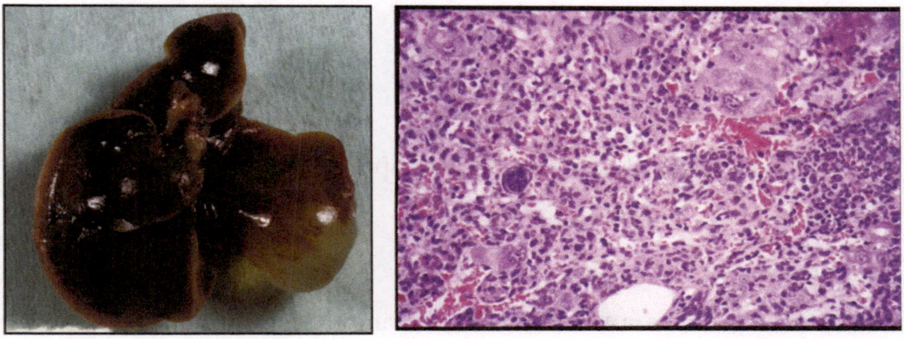

Fig. 12.1: Necrotic hepatitis in mouse

Etiology

- *Clostridium piliforme*
- Gram positive, Spore forming, Anaerobe

Pathogenesis

- Horizontal transmission- faecal oral route
- Contaminated feed, water
- Bacteria in gut causing enteritis

- Reaches liver leading to necrotic hepatitis
- Death occurs within few days of infection

Clinical manifestations

- Watery diarrhoea, dehydration, emaciation
- Occasional melena

Macroscopic features

- Hemorrhagic enteritis involving ileum, caecum and colon.
- Greyish yellow necrotic lesions on liver, heart.

Microscopic features

- Degeneration, necrosis and hemorrhage in intestines.
- Necrosis, infiltration of neutrophils and mononuclear cells in liver and heart.

Diagnosis

- Symptoms and lesions.
- Demonstration of Bacteria in liver impression Smear.
- Isolation of bacteria from liver.

Pseudotuberculosis

Pseudotuberculosis is a disease of mice, rats, G.pigs and rabbits caused by *Corynebaeterium pseudotuberculosis* and characterized by the presence of caseative nodules on lungs, kidneys, liver etc.

Etiology

- *Corynebacterium pseudotuberculosis*
- Gram positive, rods, pleomorphic.

Pathogenesis

- Direct contact
- Sub clinical infection
- Oral cavity and cervical lymph node
- Stress, immunosuppression may lead to lung infection.

- Nodule formations in lungs.

Clinical Manifestations

- Subclinical infection
- Rough hair coat, anorexia, abnormal posture.
- Dyspnoea, occulo-nasal discharge.

Macroscopic factures

- Pyogranulomatous lesions in lungs, liver, kidney.

Microscopic features

- Caseative necrosis with infiltration of neutrophils, macrophages, lymphocytes, epithelial cells and Giant cells.
- Presence of Gram positive short rods in the centre of lesions.

Diagnosis

- Symptoms and Lesions
- Presence of Gram positive short rods.
- Impression smears of the lesion - demonstration of bacteria.

Salmonellosis

Salmonellosis is an infectious bacterial disease of laboratory animals including rats, mice and rabbits and characterized by fever, diarrhoea, multifocal necrotic foci on liver.

Etiology

- *Salmonella enterica*
- Gram negative, rods.

Pathogenesis

- Transmission is through faecal oral route.
- Vertical Transmission.
- Cause sub clinical infections.

Clinical Manifestations

- Sub clinical infection.
- Diarrhoea, dehydration.
- Weight loss, conjunctivitis.

Macroscopic features

- Splenomegaly.
- Multi focal necrotic foci on liver, Kidney, spleen and intestines.

Microscopic features

- Necrosis.
- Infiltration of neutrophils, macrophages, lymphocytes.
- Lesions more pronounced in liver, Spleen, Kidneys.

Diagnosis

- Symptoms and lesions.
- Cultural examination from liver.
- Impression Smear – Gram's staining demonstration of Gram negative rods.

Infectious ectromelia

Infectious ectromelia is also known as mouse pox. It is an infectious disease of mice caused by Poxvirus and characterized by facial oedema, pustules on skin, ulcers on muzzle, limbs, ears, and tail (Fig.12.2).

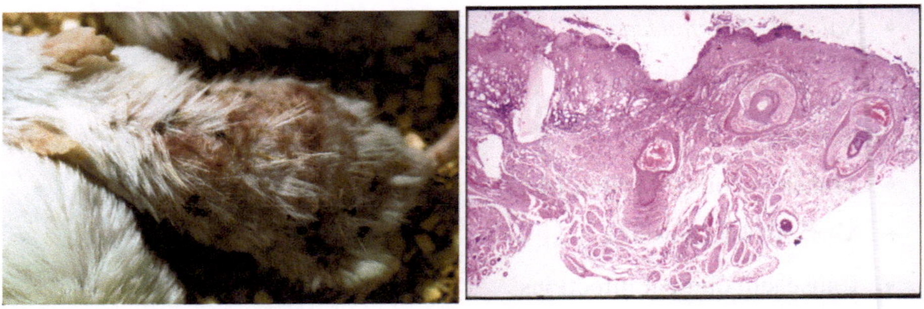

Fig. 12.2: Infectious ectromelia in mouse- **1.** Pustules on skin and **2.** Hydropic degeneration, vesicles and eosinophilic intracytoplasmic inclusions.

Etiology

- Poxvirus – Mouse pox.
- DNA virus of Poxviridae family.

Pathogenesis

- Transmission - direct contact.
- Fomites, cutaneous trauma.
- Causes pock lesions on skin within 7-11 days.
- Animal handlers may also transmit the disease.

Clinical Manifestations

- Facial oedema, swelling of legs.
- Conjunctivitis.
- Cutaneous pustules.
- Ulcer on muzzle, legs, ears, tail.
- Ectromelia – partial amputation of limbs or tail.

Macroscopic features

- Necrotic foci on lever.
- Pustules on skins.
- Ulcers on ears, legs, tail.

Microscopic features

- Hepatocellular necrosis
- Necrosis in Spleen, Thymus, Peyer's patches.
- Pustules and ulcers on Skin.
- Intracytoplasmic eosinophilic inclusions.

Diagnosis

- Symptoms and lesions
- Intracytoplasmic inclusions in cutaneous lesion - smears/ sections.
- Virus isolation/ demonstration, PCR.

Infantile diarrhoea

Infantile diarrhoea is an infectious viral disease of mice caused by rotavirus and characterized by watery, yellowish diarrhoea in baby mice below 2 weeks of age. This disease is also known as epizootic diarrhoea of infant mice (EDIM) (Fig.12.3).

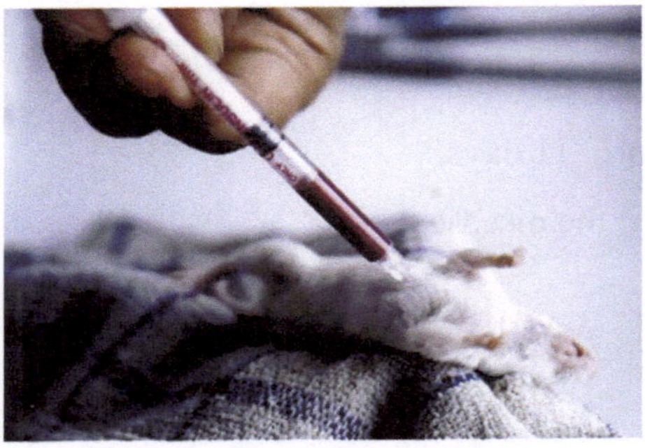

Fig. 12.3. Collection of blood from heart of mouse suffering from diarrhoea due to rotavirus infection for immunological assays.

Etiology

- Rotavirus
- Double stranded RNA, 11 Segments

Pathogenesis

- Virus is highly contagious
- Transmission through contact, beddings, fomites
- Epitheliotropic virus settles in gut epithelium.
- *Mal digestion, mal absorption, desquamation of* small intestine epithelium.

Clinical manifestations

- Diarrhoea, - watery, yellowish in 1– 14 day mice
- Lethargy
- Distended abdomen

Macroscopic features

- Watery yellowish intestinal content
- Impaction of rectum.

Microscopic features

- Atrophy of villi, fusion of villi
- Decreased absorptive surface
- Infiltration of mononuclear cells.

Diagnosis

- Symptoms & Lesions
- Demonstrationofvirusisdesquamatedcellsusing IFT/immunoperoxidase techniques.

Murine Hepatitis

Murine hepatitis is a viral disease of mice caused by coronavirus and characterized by focal necrotic hepatitis (Fig.12.4).

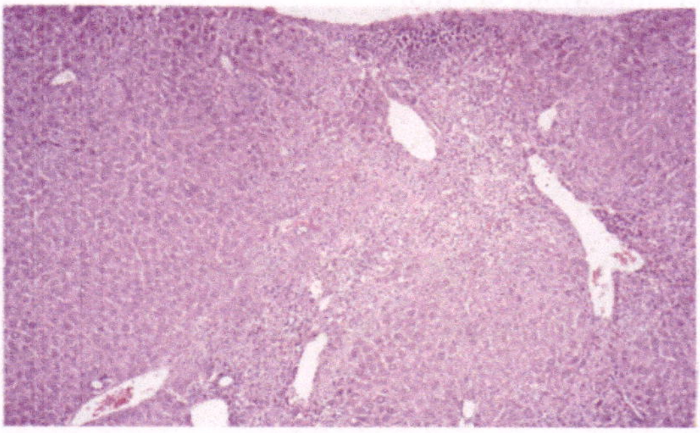

Fig. 12.4: Necrotic hepatitis

Etiology

- Corona virus.
- RNA virus, Single stranded.
- Common contaminant of Cell cultures

Pathogenesis

- Infection Spreads though aerosol, fomites and contact.
- Virus replicates in respiratory mucosa, then leads to viraemia and finally settles in liver causing necrotic lesions.
- May go to intestinal tract causing formation of syncytia in crypts.

Clinical manifestations

- Mostly asymptomatic.
- Diarrhoea.
- Dysentery.

Microscopic features

- Multifocal necrotic hepatitis.
- Enteritis – catarrhal and /or hemorrhagic.
- Presence of desquamated cells in intestinal contents.

Microscopic features

- Necrosis in liver.
- Syncytia formation in liver, intestinal crypts.
- Necrotic lesions in lymph nodes.

Diagnosis

- Symptoms and lesions.
- Demonstration of syncytia in liver and crypts of colon and caecum.
- Demonstration of virus using IFT/ Immunoperoxidase.

Lymphocytic choriomeningitis

Lymphocytic choriomeningitis is a viral disease of mice and hamsters caused by arenavirus and characterized by lymphocytic choriomeningitis, immune complex mediated glomerulonephritis and vasculitis (Fig.12.5).

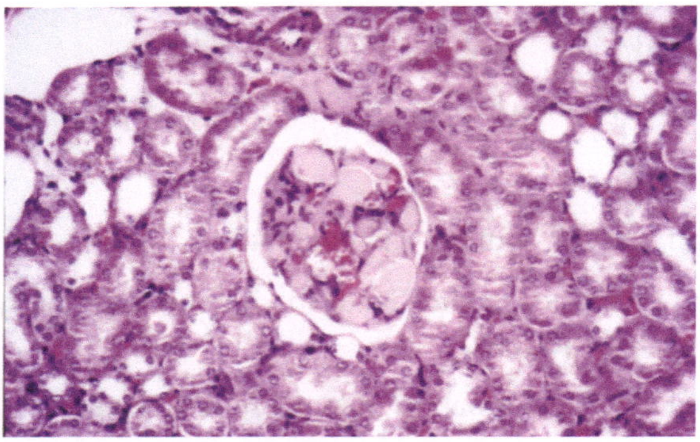

Fig. 12.5: Lymphoctic choriomeningitis –glomerulonephritis and vasculitis in kidney.

Etiology

- Arena virus
- RNA virus

Pathogenesis

- Reservoir of the virus is mice; most rodents are sensitive to infection.
- Rats are naturally resistant.
- Transmissions though contact with saliva, nasal secretions and /or urine.
- *In utero* transmission also occurs in mice.
- Persistent subclinical infection leading to immune complex mediated problems.

Clinical manifestations

- Nasal discharge.
- Proteinurea.

Macroscopic features

- Congestion of meninges and /or brain.
- Enlargement of kidneys.

Microscopic features

- Lymphocytic Choriomeningitis.
- Vasculitis.
- Immune complex mediated glomerulonephritis.
- Lymphocytic infiltration in Kidneys.

Diagnosis

- Symptoms and lesions.
- Demonstration of virus using IFT/ immunoperoxidase.

Pasteurellosis

Pasteurellosis is an infectious disease of rabbits caused by *Pasteurella* Spp and characterized by nasal discharge, pneumonia, conjunctivitis and torticollis. It is also known as snuffles.

Etiology

- *Pasteurella multocida*, normal inhabitant of upper respiratory tract.
- Gram negative, Bipolar.
- Stress is main predisposing factor.

Pathogeneses

- Transmission occurs through contact, fighting and mating.
- Infection spreads in upper respiratory tract.
- Infected rabbit acts as carriers.
- Causes nasal discharge, catarrhal rhinitis.
- Pneumonia.

Clinical Manifestations

- Nasal discharge.
- Sneezing, congestion on face.
- conjunctivitis, excess tearing, otitis media.

Macroscopic features

- Conjunctivitis
- Oedema and congestion on face.
- Pneumonia, rhinitis.
- Congestion of uterus.

Microscopic features

- Serofibrinous pneumonia.
- Congestion and haemorrhage in lymph node, spleen.
- Organism in nasal discharge.

Diagnosis

- Symptoms and lesions.
- Demonstration of bipolar bacteria.
- Isolation of bacteria.

Treponematosis

Treponematosis is a sexually transmissible disease of rabbits caused by *Treponema* spp and characterized by abortion, vulvitis, vaginitis and cervicitis in females and posthitis in males (Fig.12.6).

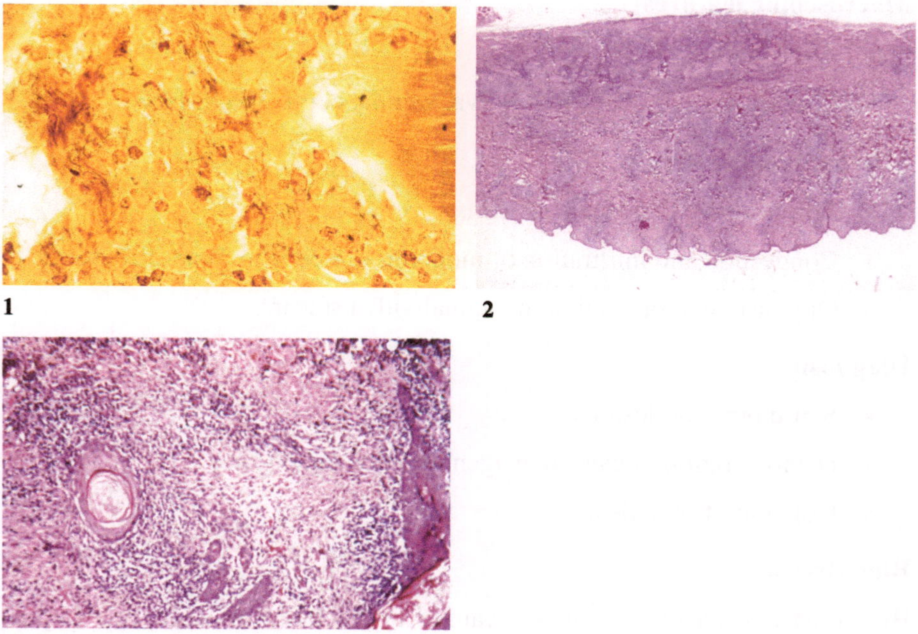

1 2

3

Fig.12.6: Chronic posthitis in rabbit due to Treponema cuniculi 1. Presence of spirochaete in silver stained section, 2. Proliferative lesions and 3. Proliferation of fibroblasts and infiltration of mononuclear cells in skin of prepuce.

Etiology

- *Treponema paraluis cuniculi.*
- Spirochaete.

Pathogenesis

- Infections spreads through coitus, contact.
- Congenital infection *in utero* or during parturition.
- Infection sets in genital organs causing abortion, vulvitis, vaginitis and cervicitis.

Clinical manifestations

- Swelling and redness of vulva, lips, and nose.
- Abortions, Long and difficult deliveries.

Macroscopic features

- Abortion
- Congestion and oedema of vulva, vagina, cervix, nose, face.

Microscopic features

- Congestion and oedema of skin.
- Congestion and infiltration of mononuclear cells in liver of foetus.
- Organism demonstration in vaginal/vulva smears.

Diagnosis

- Symptoms and lesions.
- Demonstration of causative agent in vulvular smears.
- Isolation of organism.

Blue Breast

Blue breast is mastitis in rabbits, caused by bacterial infection due to poor sanitation and characterized by hot, red, swollen, cyanotic mammary glands. It is also known as 'blue bag'.

Etiology

- *Staphylococcus aureus*.
- *Streptococcus pyogenes*.
- Many other infections.

Pathogenesis

- Poor sanitation and unhygienic conditions.
- Teat canal infection.
- Bacteria enters in mammary gland causes inflammation.
- Cyanosis of mammary gland **blue bag**.

Clinical manifestations

- Fever
- Red, hot, Swollen and painful mammary gland.
- Blue breast due to cyanosis.

Microscopic features

- Blood trough teat canal.
- Acute inflammatory changes in mammary gland.

Diagnosis

- Symptoms & Lesions.
- Isolation of bacteria, causative organisms.

Enterotoxaemia

Enterotoxaemia is an infectious disease of rabbits caused by *Clostridium perfringens* type E and characterized by diarrhoea, haemorrhagic enteritis and death.

Etiology

- *Clostridium perfringens* type E - Iota Toxin.
- Gram positive rods.

Pathogenesis

- Bacteria is normal inhabitant of gut.
- Antibiotic therapy or overfeeding leads to development of toxins.
- Death occurs due to extensive blood loss.

Clinical Manifestations

- Diarrhoea, melena.
- Sudden onset of disease.
- After over feeding or Antibiotic treatment.
- Death.

Macroscopic features

- Congestion in stomach and intestines.
- Hemorrhagic enteritis.
- Endocardial haemorrhage.

Microscopic features

- Necrotic erosive or ulcerative typhlitis.
- Sub mucosal oedema and haemorrhage.
- Bacteria can be seen on mucosal surface.

Diagnosis

- Symptoms and lesions.
- Demonstration of Bactria.
- Detections of iota toxins in intestinal contents.

Rabbit Pox

Rabbit Pox is an infectious viral disease of rabbits caused by orthopox virus and characterized by the presence of pock lesions on skin, subcutaneous oedema and oedema of mouth.

Etiology

- Rabbit pox virus
- DNA virus of Poxviridae family.

Pathogenesis

- Airborne infection rapidly spreads.
- Causes subcutaneous oedema.
- High rate of mortality.

Clinical Manifestations

- Pock lesions may or may not present on skin.
- Subcutaneous oedema, facial oedema.
- Fever, nasal discharge, Skin rashes.
- High Mortality.

Macroscopic features

- Subcutaneous and facial oedema.
- Pock lesions.
- Sometimes pox less rabbit pox- confused with myxomatosis.

Microscopic features

- Subcutaneous oedema.
- Intracytoplasmic eosinophilic inclusions in skin epithelial cells.
- Infiltration of mononuclear cells.

Diagnosis

- Symptoms and lesions.
- Isolation of virus / Demonstration of inclusion bodies.
- Serology to differentiate myxomatosis.

Infectious myxomatosis

Infectious myxomatosis is a viral disease of rabbits caused by myxoma virus and characterized by skin tumors, lumps and puffiness around head and genitalia.

Etiology

- Myxoma virus of leporipoxvirus group - family Poxviridae.
- Ds DNA virus.

Pathogenesis

- Disease Spreads through direct contact
- Mechanical transmission by fleas, mosquitoes.
- Development of skin tumors.
- Secondary bacterial infection may lead to suppurative pneumonia.

Clinical Manifestations

- Fever, conjunctivitis.
- Puffiness around head and genitalia.

- Skin tumors.
- Nasal discharge.

Macroscopic features

- Skin tumors.
- Puffiness around head and genitalia.
- Suppurative pneumonia.

Microscopic features

- Hyperplasia, anaplasia and neoplastic cells in skin.
- Intracytoplasmic inclusions (sometimes).

Diagnosis

- Symptoms and lesions.
- Demonstration of virus/isolation.
- Serology.

Papillomatosis

Papillomatosis is a viral disease of rabbits caused by Papilloma virus and characterized by the development of small, wart like growth papilloma over the skin.

Etiology

- Shope Papilloma virus.
- Oral Papilloma virus.

Pathogenesis

- Infection Spreads through contact, insects.
- Causes skin infection – hyperplasia of stratum spinosum layer of skin.
- Shope papilloma also known as **cotton tail papilloma**.

Clinical Manifestations

- Development of raised, red, rough lesions on skin of neck, shoulders, eyelids, ears.
- Oral papilloma occurs on tongue and oral mucosa.

Macroscopic features

- Presence of papilloma on skin.
- Presence of Papilloma on oral wily.
- Ulceration, sloughing and re-epitheliazation.

Microscopic features

- Hyperplasia of skin epithelium particularly in stratum spinosum layer.
- Ulceration, re-epitheliazation.

Diagnosis

- Symptoms and lesions.
- Demonstration of the virus.
- Isolation of the virus.

Coccidiosis

Coccidiosis is a protozoan parasitic disease of rabbits caused by different Species of *Eimeria* spp and characterized by intestinal and hepatic lesions (Fig.12.7).

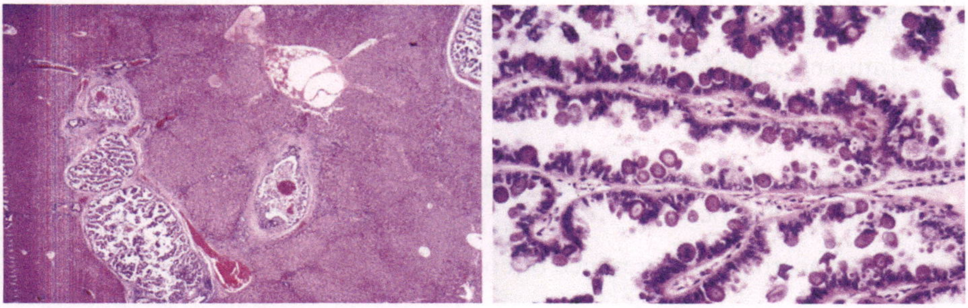

Fig. 12.7: Hepatic coccidiosis in rabbit 1. Bile duct hyperplasia and ectasia and 2. Presence of coccidia parasites in liver section.

Etiology

Intestinal coccidiosis

- *Eimeria perforans*
- *E. magna*
- *E. media*
- *E. irresidua*

Hepatic coccidiosis

- *E. steidae*

Pathogenesis

- Contagious protozoan parasite spreads through contact, ingestion – fecal oral route.
- Invade the epithelial cells of intestinal wall.
- Hepatic coccidia invade the cells of bile duct and liver causing blockage and severe liver damage.

Clinical manifestations

- Rough coat, dullness, weight loss, dehydration.
- Convulsions, Paralysis.
- Pot belly in hepatic form.
- Diarrhoea, melena.

Macroscopic features

- Hemorrhage in intestines.
- Small focal necrotic foci on liver.
- Intussusception – telescoping of intestines.

Microscopic features

- Necrosis in intestinal epithelium with presence of hemorrhage and intracellular coccidia.
- Liver necrosis and presence of coccidia.

Diagnosis

- Symptoms and lesions.
- Demonstration of coccidia in stool, intestinal scrapings and liver impression smears.

Mite infestation (Mange)

Mange is parasitic disease of rabbits caused by mites and characterize by ear infestation, fur infestation (cheyletiellosis) and burrowing in skin by mites.

Etiology

1. Ear mites – *Psoroptes cuniculi*
2. Fur mites – *Cheyletiella parasitovorax, Listrophorus gibbus*
3. Burrowing miles – *Sarcoptes scabiei*

Pathogenesis

- Infection spreads through contact, fomites.
- Mite infests skin causing lesions.

Clinical Manifestation

- Ear mange – ear, head, neck, legs, ventral portion of abdomen- scratching, inflammatory lesions, skin scales.
- Fur mites – on keratin layer of skin on dorsum and neck producing dandruff and increased secretion of fatly matter (Seborrheic lesions).
- Mange – scabies – by hyper keratinization of skin, scratching wounds.

Macroscopic features

- Increased skin thickness.
- Otitis externa.
- Presence of mites in fur leading to seborrheic lesions.

Microscopic features

- Hyperplasia and hyper keratinization of skin epithelium.
- Presence of mites in lesion.
- Congestion and hemorrhage in skin.

Diagnosis

- Symptoms and lesions.
- Demonstration of mites in skin scraping examination.

13

Pathology of Wild Animal Diseases

Feline Leukemia

Feline leukemia is an infectious viral disease of cats, lion, tiger etc. caused by oncorna virus and characterized by malignant lymphoma, lymphocytosis and immunosuppression. It is also known as feline lymphoma or feline lymphosarcoma.

Etiology

- Oncorna virus of retroviridae family
- Type C oncorna virus, RNA virus has reverse transcriptase

Pathogenesis

The virus is transmitted horizontally through salivary and nasal secretions of sick cats. It affects lymphocytes causing their proliferation leading to production of neoplastic growth.

Characteristic symptoms

- Enlargement of superficial lymph nodes
- Lymphocytosis
- Chronic diarrhoea
- Abortion

Macroscopic features

- Enlargement of lymph nodes (mesenteric, lumbar)
- Enteritis
- Anemia
- Placentitis

Microscopic features

- Lymphocytosis
- Anaplastic lymphoid cells in lymph nodes

Diagnosis

- Symptoms and lesions
- Detection of viral antigen/antibody using ELISA
- Demonstration of viral antigen using immunoperoxidase technique
- Demonstration of virus using electronmicroscopy

Feline panleukopenia

Feline panleukopenia is a viral disease of cats caused by feline parvovirus and characterised by panleukopenia, bloody diarrhoea, severe dehydration, anemia and often fatal.

Etiology

- Feline parvovirus
- A close relative of canine parvovirus

Pathogenesis

- Spreads through contact
- Bedding, food dishes, clothing and shoes of handlers of infected animals
- Fleas
- Extremely resistant
- Attacks the lining of the gastrointestinal tract
- Ulceration and sloughing of the intestinal epithelium
- Bloody diarrhoea, severe dehydration, anemia, and often death

Characteristic symptoms

- Decrease in the cat's white blood cells
- Panleukopenia
- Diphasic Fever
- Vomiting

- Dehydration
- Self-biting in the tail, lower back and back legs
- Death

Macroscopic features

- Panleukopenia
- Cerebellar hypoplasia
- Haemorrhagic enteritis
- Ulcers in intestines
- Myocarditis

Microscopic features

- Desquamation of intestinal epithelium
- Hemorrhage
- Ulceration
- Intra nuclear inclusions in intestinal epithelial cells

Myocarditis

Diagnosis

- Symptoms and lesions
- Detection of viral antigen/antibody using ELISA
- Demonstration of viral antigen using immunoperoxidase technique
- Demonstration of virus using electronmicroscopy

West Nile fever

West Nile fever is an infectious viral disease of wild animals and birds caused by flavi virus and characterized by stumbling, twitching of muscles, partial paralysis, coma and death. If can spreads to human beings also.

Etiology

- West Nile virus of Flaviviridae family
- RNA virus, insect – vectors

Pathogenesis

- Primary host of west nile virus - wild birds
- Mosquito spreads the virus among birds
- Incidental host – equines, man.
- Viremia, fever, nervous signs.

Clinical manifestations

- Fever, flu like symptoms in man.
- Muscle twitching, blindness
- Partial or complete paralysis
- Coma and death

Macroscopic features

- Congestion of meninges and brain
- Necrotic foci in brain.
- Muscle necrosis.

Microscopic features

- Encephalitis – perivascular tufting.
- Necrosis of nervous tissue.
- Mononuclear cell infiltration.
- Microglial cells proliferation and nodule formation.

Diagnosis

- Symptoms and lesions.
- Demonstration of viral antigen in nervous tissue using IFT. Immunoperoxidase techniques.
- Detection of antibodies/antigen through ELIISA.

Rabies

Rabies is an infectious viral disease of wild animals caused by lyssa virus and characterized by nervous signs, encephalitis and intra cytoplasmic eosinophilic inclusions in brain cells. Wild animals include: Fox, Wolf, cat, monkey, mongoose, rabbit etc (Fig.13.1).

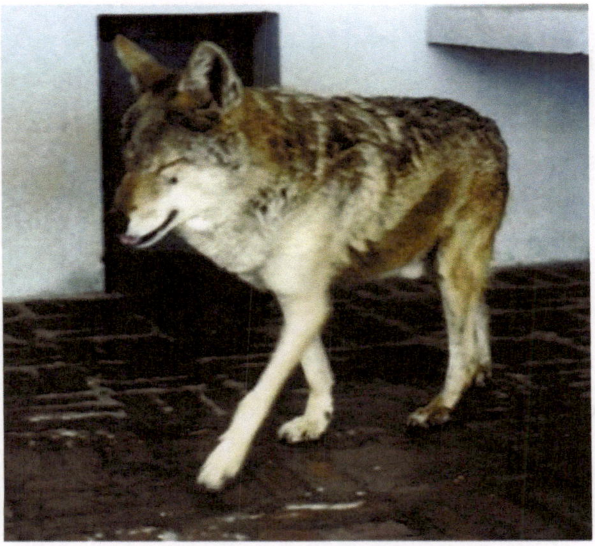

Fig. 13.1:

Etiology

- Rhabdoviridae family – Lyssavirus
- Bullet shaped, RNA virus.

Pathogenesis

- Spreads through bite of animals.
- Virus multiply in muscles, reaches in motor end plates in nerves.
- Reaches brain though centripetal force 3-4 mm/hr.
- Causes encephalitis, through nerves virus reaches to salivary glands.
- Excretes out in saliva even before onset of symptoms.

Clinical manifestations

- Aim less movement.
- Pica- eating of non- food materials.
- Nervous signs – paralysis, death.

Macroscopic features

- No characteristic lesion.
- Encephalitis.
- Non - food items in stomach.
- Presence of bite wound on skin.

Microscopic features

- Congestion in brain.
- Perivascular cuffing of mononuclear cells.
- Presence of intra cytoplasmic eosinophilic inclusions -**Negri bodies**.

Diagnosis

- Symptoms and lesions.
- Presence of Intra cytoplasmic eosinophilic inclusions in brain cells.
- Immunofluorescence test or mice inoculation test.

Foot and Mouth disease

Foot and mouth disease is an infectious viral disease of wild animals caused by picorna virus and Characterized by fever, presence of vesicles on oral mucosa and foot. Wild animals include: Deer, Wild boars, Bison, Wild buffalo, Mithun, Gaur, Elephant.

Etiology

- Picornavirus of Picornaviridae.
- RNA virus – Seven serotypes – O, A, C, Asia – 1, SAT-1, SAT-2, SAT-3.

Pathogenesis

- Transmission – Inhalation, ingestion, inoculation fomites.
- Virus replicates in pharynx.
- Viremia, epitheliotropic virus – epithelium of mouth.
- Viral excretion 24hr prior to the onset of disease.

Characteristic Symptoms

- Fever (102-104°F).
- Drooling of Saliva.
- Vesicles in mouth cavity and foot.
- Lameness.

Macroscopic features

- Vesicles in month cavity.
- Vesicles in coronet of foot.
- In young ones – necrotic myocarditis.

Microscopic features

- Vesicles in oral mucosa, tongue.
- Infiltration of mononuclear cells.
- Congestion, hemorrhage, necrosis of cardiac muscles.

Diagnosis

- Symptoms and lesions
- Demonstration of virus is salivary secretions/vesicular fluid.
- Isolation of the virus.

Kyasanur Forest Disease (KFD)

Kyasanur forest disease is an infectious viral disease of wild animals and characterized by fever, myalgia, coughing, diarrhea, vomiting and photophobia. It mostly occurs in Langur, Monkeys, Rats, Shrews, and can cause disease in man.

Etiology

- Flavirus of flaviviridae family.
- Ticks – intermediate host.

Pathogenesis

- Virus transmitted through ticks in small mammals like rats and in ground birds.

- Monkeys get infected trough ticks.
- Human beings get infected while visit /pass through forest area - by the bite of nymph of ticks.

Clinical manifestations

- Fever, relapsed after 1-2 weeks.
- Headache, myalgia, coughing, diarrhea.
- Neck stiffness.
- Photophobia.
- Death.

Macroscopic features

- Stiffness of muscles.
- Enteritis.
- Necrosis of muscles.
- Congestion in meninges and brain.

Microscopic features

- Necrosis of myofibrils.
- Hemorrhagic gastroenteritis.
- Congestion of brain.
- Infiltration of mononuclear cells.

Diagnosis

- Symptoms and lesions.
- Detection of virus in animals and ticks.
- Isolation of the virus.

Infectious hepatitis

Infectious hepatitis is a viral disease of wild animals caused by hepatitis E virus and characterized by icterus and hepatitis. It causes disease in wild boar, deer, and accidentally in man.

Etiology

- Hepatitis E virus of herpesviridae family.
- DNA virus.

Pathogenesis

- Spreads through contact, ingestion of contaminated food and water.
- Reaches liver – causing hepatopathy.
- Leads to icterus, vomiting, diarrhoea.

Clinical Manifestation

- Vomiting, diarrhoea, fever.
- Icterus – mucous membrane of oral cavity – yellow.
- Dark yellow urine.
- Weakness, death.

Macroscopic features

- Necrosis, Congestion and hemorrhage in liver.
- Icterus.
- Gastroenteritis.

Microscopic features

- Necrotic hepatitis.
- Gastroenteritis.
- Lymphadenopathy.

Diagnosis

- Symptoms and lesions.
- Icterus.
- Demonstration of virus /antigen in clinical specimens.

Pox

Pox is an infectious viral disease of wild animals caused by members of poxviridae family and characterized by the presence of pock lesions on hair less parts of the skin. It causes disease in wild mammals (Squirrels, rabbits, cats, zebra, monkeys, bison. Fox etc.) as well as in wild birds (Pigeons, parrots, pheasants, quails, wild turkeys etc.) (Fig.13.2).

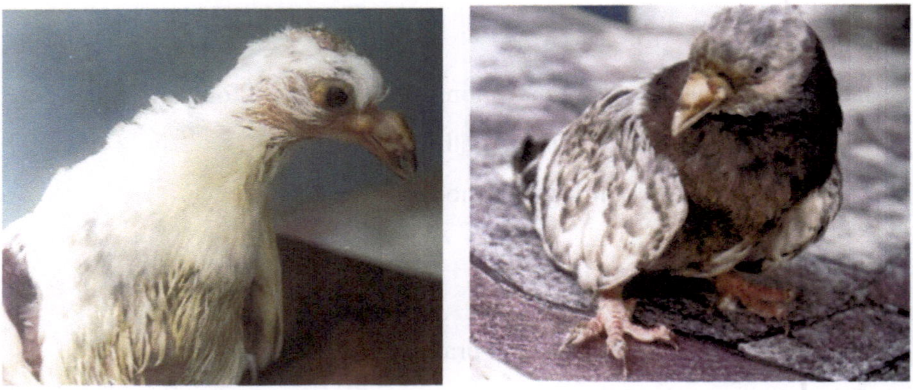

Fig. 13.2: Pox in pigeons- Pock lesions on beak and claws.

Etiology

- Pox virus of poxviridae family
- DNA virus, largest virus

Pathogenesis

- Disease is transmitted by direct contact with affected animals and insects.
- Virus enters through small abrasions of skin.
- Incubation period of 3-7 days.
- Pock lesions appear on skin - erythema, papules, vesicles, pustule and scab.
- On detach and slough off lesions may leave scar.

Characteristic symptoms

- Fever (105-107°F)
- Pock lesions on hairless parts of skin like papule, vesicle, pustule, scab and scar

Macroscopic features

- Presence of pock lesions on hair less parts of body including papule, vesicle, pustule, scab and scar.
- Pock lesions on teats, face, whole body

Microscopic features

- Necrosis of stratum spinosum epithelium of epidermis
- Infiltration of mononuclear cells in dermis and epidermis
- Presence of intracytoplasmic inclusions

Diagnosis

- Symptoms and lesions
- Immunodiagnostic tests for demonstration of antigen /antibody
- AGPT
- ELISA
- Isolation of virus

Tuberculosis

Tuberculosis is a chronic bacterial disease of wild animals caused by *Mycobacterium* sp. and characterized by presence of tubercle nodules in lungs, spleen and lymph nodes (Fig.13.3).

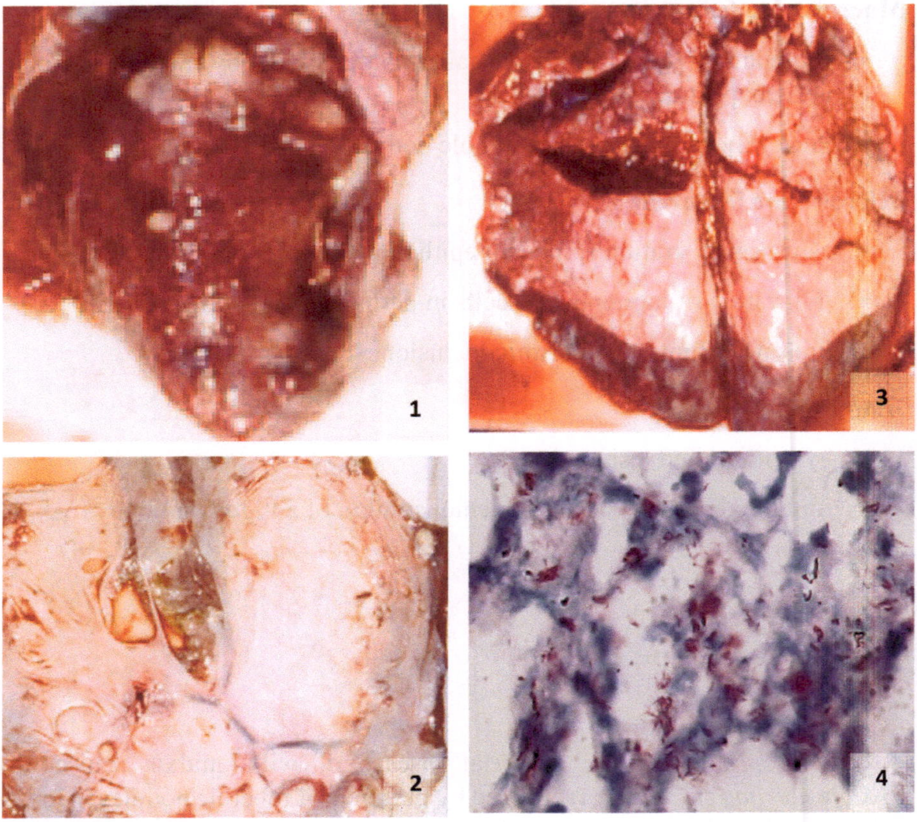

Fig. 13 3: Tuberculosis in deer- (1) Tuberculous nodules on epicardium, (2) diaphragm, (3) lungs, and (4) acid-fast bacilli in lung tissue section

Etiology

- *Mycobacterium tuberculosis*
- *M. bovis*

Pathogenesis

Disease spreads through contact with infected animals or their discharges or morbid tissues. The infected animals release the organisms through sputum at coughing and contact animals get infection through droplet inhalation. Besides sputum, faeces, urine, vaginal discharges, semen, milk, lymph and wound discharges may act source of infection. It is also transmitted through contaminated instruments, utensils and beddings. After entry through inhalation or ingestion, bacilli localizes at the point of entry and produce typical tubercle in associated lymph nodes. Mostly pharyngeal and mesenteric lymph nodes are affected. From lymph nodes, infection may extend across body cavities, blood vessels and lymph vessels. The inhaled organism enter in the bronchial tree after lodging in bronchi a tissue reaction takes place. Neutrophilic infiltration is there and when neutrophils are necrosed, macrophages come to destroy the organism but they fail then many macrophages becomes elongated to form epithelioid cells, the hall mark of granulomatous inflammation. Some macrophages are joint together to form giant cells to destroy the acid fast bacilli. As a consequence of this some bacilli are phagocytosed and are destroyed. A zone of lymphocytes, macrophages, epithelioid cells, giant cells and fibrous connective tissues are formed around the central necrosed area.

Characteristic symptoms

- Low grade fever
- Progressive wasting/weakness, loss of production
- Coughing

Macroscopic features

- Consolidation of lungs
- Nodules of tubercle present in lungs containing cheesy mass
- Granulomatous lesions in spleen, lymph nodes, liver and intestines.
- Tubercle on pleura and mesentery (***pearly disease***).

Microscopic features

- Granulomatous lesions characterized by the presence of tubercles in different organs
- Tubercle consists of central caseative necrosed area surrounded by macrophages, lymphocytes, epithelioid cells and giant cells
- In older cases central necrosed area is calcified and surrounded by fibrous tissue capsule.

Diagnosis

- Symptoms and lesions
- Tuberculin testing of animals
- Immunodiagnostic tests for demonstration of antigen /antibody
- ELISA

- Demonstration of acid fast bacilli in impression smears of tubercle or in tissue sections of lungs and lymph nodes.

Braxy

Braxy is an acute fatal disease of wild ruminents like deer caused by *Clostridium septicum* and characterized by oedema, necrosis and haemorrhage in abomasum (Fig.13.4).

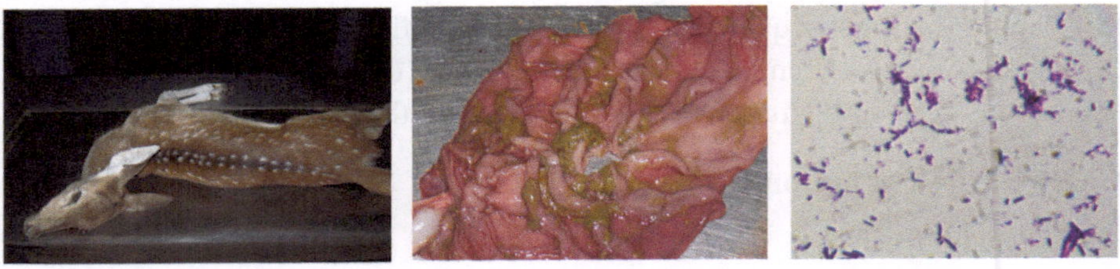

Fig. 13.4: Braxy in deer. 1. Dead deer, 2. Oedematous and congested abomasum and 3. Clostrdium septicum

Etiology

- *Clostridium septicum*

Pathogenesis

It is a soil borne infection and mostly occurs in sheep vaccinated with enterotoxaemia vaccine. The organism gets entry through ingestion of spores. The ingested spores are localized in stomach and germinate under anaerobic conditions due to over feeding of lush green feed or high amount of grains leading to abomasitis.

Characteristic symptoms

- Over filled stomach
- Sudden mortality
- History of enterotoxaemia vaccination

Macroscopic features

- Oedema of abomasal folds
- Congestion and haemorrhage in abomasum
- Necrosis of abomasal mucosa
- Congestion and necrosis in intestines.

Microscopic features

- Congestion and haemorrhage of abomasal mucosa
- Presence of 'Rod' shaped organism in mucosal epithelium of abomasum
- Necrosis and presence of ulcers in abomasal mucosa.

Diagnosis

- History of over feeding and enterotoxaemia vaccination
- Symptoms and lesions
- Demonstration of toxin in intestinal/ stomach contents on mouse inoculation test
- Isolation and identification of bacteria

Colibacillosis

Colibacillosis is an infectious disease of new born animals caused by *E. coli* and characterized by enteritis, swelling of lymph nodes and peyer's patches, pneumonia and haemorrhage on endocardium.

Etiology

- *Escherichia coli*

Pathogenesis

The disease is transmitted through contaminated feed and water. Discharges of aborted foetus, vaginal discharges, umbilical infection and intrauterine infection may act as source of infection for newly born animals. The colonization of organism in gut depends on the immune status animals. The cell wall of *E.coli* consists of lipopolysaccharide which causes fever mediated through the production of host cytokines including TNF and IL-1. *E.coli* also secretes substances that suppresses phagocytosis by neutrophils. The endotoxins secreted by *E.coli* is an ADP- ribosyltransferase which generate excess c- AMP to cause diarrhoea and dehydration.

Characteristic symptoms

- Fever(103-106°F)
- Diarrhoea, dehydration
- Nasal discharges
- Naval ill

Macroscopic features

- Swollen umblicus
- Swelling of joints
- Suppurative nephritis
- Congestion and haemorrhage in intestines
- Congestion of lungs and mesenteric lymph nodes
- Haemorrhage in endocardium.

Microscopic features

- Necrosis and desquamation of mucosal epithelium in intestine
- Infiltration of neutrophils and mononuclear cells
- Infiltration of neutrophils in kidneys forming micro abscess
- Catarrhal bronchopneumonia
- Congestion and reactive hyperplasia in lymph nodes.

Diagnosis

- Symptoms and lesions
- Isolation of bacteria
- Immunodiagnostic tests for demonstration of antigen /antibody
- ELISA
- Demonstration of organisms in tissue sections using special stains.

Anthrax

Anthrax is an acute septicemic disease of animals caused by *Bacillus* sp. and characterized by sudden death, absence of rigor mortis, tary colour blood from natural openings and widespread hemorrhage.

Etiology

- *Bacillus anthracis*

Pathogenesis

The infection occurs through ingestion or inhalation of spores/ vegetative forms of the organism or entry of bacteria through broken skin. After entry the spores germinate and localize for multiplication and spread by means of lymphatics to lymph nodes and then in blood stream, causing severe septicaemia. The bacteria possesses both capsule and exotoxin. Due to presence of capsule phagocytic cells become unable to destroy them. The exotoxin is lethal in nature, it causes oedema and tissue damage. The exotoxin has 3 components-

1. Oedema factor (EF) or factor I is adenyl cyclase which causes increase in cellular c-AMP level that causes electrolyte and fluid loss.
2. Protective antigen (PA) or factor II is a fragment of exotoxin and has anti-phagocytic activity.
3. Lethal factor (LF) or factor III stimulates macrophages for production of oxidizing radicals and cytokines. Mainly IL-1 and TNF- α, which induce shock and death.

Characteristic symptoms

- High fever(105-107°F)
- Haemorrhage from natural orifices
- Dyspnoea
- Tary colour blood
- Sudden mortality up to 90%

Macroscopic features

- Post mortem examination of animals suspected for anthrax should not be conducted.
- Blood smear examined for anthrax bacilli
- Discharge of blood from vagina, anus and mouth
- Tary colour of blood
- Enlargement of spleen
- Widespread haemorrhage on serous surfaces of visceral organs
- Subcutaneous oedema

Microscopic features

- Anthrax bacilli and spores in blood smear
- Spleen shows haemorrhage and accumulation of blood in red pulp

- Haemorrhage in lymph nodes, liver, lungs and kidneys
- Degenerative and necrotic changes in kidneys and liver.

Diagnosis

- Symptoms and lesions
- Demonstration of bacteria in blood smear
- Immunodiagnostic tests for demonstration of antigen /antibody
- ELISA
- AGPT (Ascoli test)
- Animal inoculation test causes death of mouse within 24 hrs.

Trypanosomosis

Trypanosomosis is an infectious disease of wild animals caused by protozoan parasite and characterized by emaciation, enlargement of spleen and lymph nodes, petechiae on serous membranes, ulceration on tongue and gastric mucosa and gelatinous exudate in subcutaneous region (Fig.13.5).

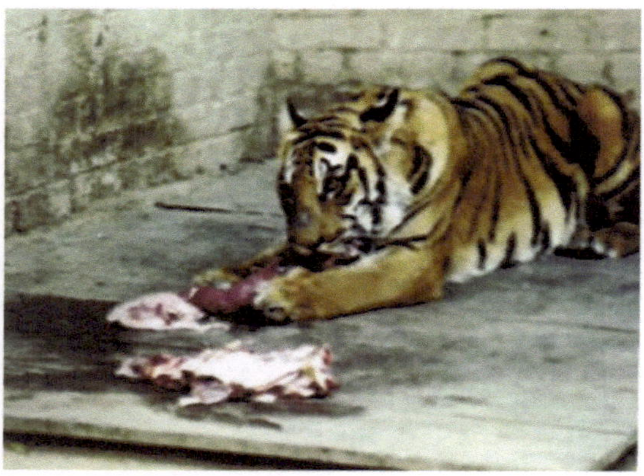

Fig. 13.5: Trypanosomosis in a tiger.

Etiology

- *Trypanosoma evansi*

Pathogenesis

The disease is mainly transmitted through bite of flies like Tabanus, Stomoxys, Haematopota etc. The carrier animals remain as potential source of infection. The pathogenesis of disease is not completely known. After entering in mammalian host, trypanosomes multiply in blood stream by binary fission leading to parasitaenia. The parasites has variable surface glycoproteins which cause continuous exposure of immune system leading to hyperplasia of spleen and lymph nodes. In chronic cases, due to formation of antigen- antibody complexes glomerulonephritis and vasculitis is seen.

Characteristic symptoms

- High fever (105-107°F)
- Dyspnoea
- Paraplegia, emaciation
- Oedema in dependent parts of body
- Conjunctivitis, keratitis

Macroscopic features

- Emaciated carcass
- Enlargement of spleen and lymph nodes
- Gelatinous exudate in subcutaneous region
- Ulcerative keratitis
- Congestion of abomasum and intestines
- Petechiae on kidneys, liver and heart
- Ulcers in tongue and abomasum.

Microscopic features

- Presence of flagellate parasite in blood smear (Fig.9.1)
- Hyperplasia of lymphoid follicles in lymph nodes and spleen
- Congestion in intestines
- Erosion and ulcers in abomasum.

Diagnosis

- Demonstration of protozoan parasite in blood smear
- Symptoms and lesions
- Immunodiagnostic tests for demonstration of antigen /antibody
- ELISA

Theileriosis

Theileriosis is an infectious disease of animals caused by protozoan parasite and characterized by enlargement of lymph nodes, pulmonary oedema, haemorrhage in kidneys and liver, ulcers in abomasum and catarrhal enteritis.

Etiology

- *Theileria annulata*

Pathogenesis

The parasite is transmitted through bite of ticks of genus Hyalomma. The disease can also be transmitted mechanically by inoculation of blood and tissue suspension made from spleen, lymph nodes and liver of infected animals. After entry the organism at sporozoit stage remains in blood circulation and enters in erythrocytes but they don't multiply. The multiplication occurs in lymphocytes where it forms schizonts. Infected lymphocytes are ruptured and schizonts are released and other lymphocytes are affected. Later some schizonts are differentiated unto merozoites. The rapidly multiplying schizonts are causing severe damage to lymphoid cells through their lysis.

Characteristic symptoms

- High fever (105-107°F)
- Anemia
- Enlargement of superficial lymph nodes

Macroscopic features

- Anemia
- Pulmonary oedema
- Enlargement of lymph nodes and spleen
- Erosions and ulcers in abomasum
- Haemorrhage in epicardium
- Catarrhal enteritis

Microscopic features

- Lymphoid depletion
- Presence of parasites in erythrocytes or its developmental stages in lymphocytes

- Perivascular lymphoid proliferation
- Congestion in intestines
- Proliferation of goblet cells.

Diagnosis

- Demonstration of protozoan parasite in blood smear/lymph node biopsy (Fig.9.2)
- Symptoms and lesions
- Immunodiagnostic tests for demonstration of antigen /antibody
- ELISA

Babesiosis

Babesiosis is an infectious disease of animals caused by protozoan parasite and characterized by hemoglobinuria, anemia, petechiae and echymosis in serous membranes, icterus, pulmonary oedema and gastroenteritis.

Etiology

- *Babesia bigemina*
- *B. bovis*

Pathogenesis

The disease is transmitted from sick to healthy animal through ticks following trans ovarian route. The incubation period of disease is 5-10 days. After infection, the parasite multiplies in peripheral blood and there is intra-vascular haemolysis leading to hemoglobinuria. The infected erythrocytes liberate some enzymes which interact with the components of blood and leads to increased erythrocyte fragility, hypertensive shock and disseminated intra ocular coagulation.

Characteristic symptoms

- High fever (105-107°F)
- Anemia, icterus
- Hemoglobinuria

Macroscopic features

- Anemia, icterus
- Hemoglobinuria
- Enlargement of spleen and liver
- Oedema in lungs
- Petechiae and echymosis in kidneys, lungs, liver and spleen
- Congestion in gastrointestinal tract

Microscopic features

- Presence of pear shaped Babesia organism in erythrocytes
- Haemorrhage in liver, kidneys, lungs and spleen
- Haemosiderosis in spleen
- Necrosis of tubular epithelium in kidneys and presence of hyaline casts.

Diagnosis

- Demonstration of protozoan parasite in blood smear (Fig.9.3)
- Symptoms and lesions
- Immunodiagnostic tests for demonstration of antigen /antibod
- ELISA

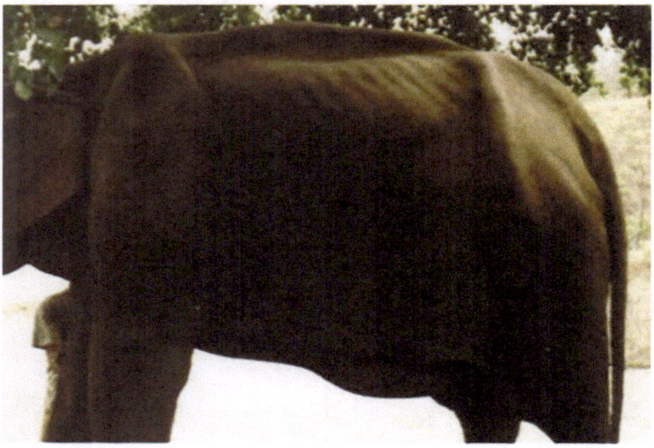

Fig. 13.6: Dropsy in an elephant.

Index

I

M

P

Q

R